Therapi
Healthy Body

For Vivienne, sister and seeker of the heart

THIS IS A CARLTON BOOK

Design copyright © 2001, 2003 Carlton Books Limited
Text copyright © 2001 Jane Alexander

This edition published by
Carlton Books Limited 2003
20 Mortimer Street, London W1T 3JW

A CIP catalogue record for this book is available from
the British Library
ISBN 1 84222 883 8

Typeset by E-Type, Liverpool
Printed and bound in England

Therapies for a Healthy Body

A Complete Guide to Holistic Therapies for
Maintaining Optimum Physical Health

Jane Alexander

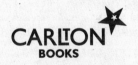
CARLTON
BOOKS

Contents

Introduction

All the information we need to have a healthier, happier, body is ours for the taking. The fields of natural healing and mind–body medicine, offer many paths to health but unfortunately we can become overwhelmed by the choice. There are literally hundreds of different therapies and teachings all promising to heal your body, in some way. Which should you choose? Where do you start? The choice can be bewildering. Fortunately, the answers lie within the pages of one book – this one.

The aim of *Therapies for a Healthy Body* is to provide a simple, straightforward, friendly guide through the maze of holistic living. We have done all the hard work for you, picking out the nuggets of sheer gold amid the tomes of heavy theory and complex philosophy. As you work your way through this clear and concise book, you will learn how to incorporate natural health into your everyday life.

I firmly believe that the most important thing any of us can do is to take responsibility for our bodies. Once we decide that we have the power to change, almost anything can happen. In the past, it has been common for many of us to hand over responsibility for our health, to other people: to doctors and hospitals; to teachers and therapists; to priests and ministers. We have relied heavily on the opinions and thoughts of other people; we have looked to newspapers, television and society for approval. Yet, when you decide that *you* are in charge of your destiny, it is almost as if a quantum leap occurs and absolutely everything is open to change.

Rest assured, you don't have to go out and make major changes overnight. Even the tiniest shift can create ripples. Adjust your diet a little, start to exercise, and you will have begun a process that almost inevitably leads to other changes. People can and do heal their bodies – so can you.

This book offers plenty of suggestions for leading healthier, life. Yet it cannot work miracles. There are times when you will need expert help. Although I have included numerous self-help tips and do-it-yourself techniques, I would strongly recommend that, if you are drawn to a particular therapy or practice, you seek out an experienced, well-qualified practitioner.

If you have any serious medical concerns or ailments, you must always see your primary care doctor. Also, be aware that some of the therapies in this book may bring past traumas or difficulties to the surface.

1 *Fundamental Principles*

Ayurveda

Ayurveda is the oldest system of medicine on earth. Its principles are said to have been passed down to humankind from a chain of gods leading back to Brahma, father of all gods. It has been called the 'mother of medicine' and is generally accepted to be the fore-runner of all the great healing systems of the world.

Written texts show that the ayurvedic medicine practised from about 1500 bc to ad 500 was incredibly advanced, with detailed knowledge of pediatrics, psychiatry, surgery, geriatrics, toxicology, general medicine and other specialties. However, invasions disrupted its teaching and, when the British introduced Western medicine to India, ayurveda became unfashionable and almost disappeared entirely. It was saved, however, by the intervention of Mahatma Gandhi who opened the first new ayurvedic college in 1921.

The fundamental aim of ayurveda is to attain perfect health and wellbeing. The ancient texts say that the human lifespan should be around 100 years – and that all those years should be lived in total health, both physical and mental. The ayurvedic practitioner is there-fore looking to balance the body and mind, to ferret out health problems before they happen or to nip them in the bud before they do any real harm. Unfortunately, illnesses (and the shortening of life) are caused by many factors: constant stress; irregular meals; eating the wrong kind of food; taking the wrong medication; living an unhealthy lifestyle; having bad body posture; breathing in polluted air; allowing microorganisms to enter the body; becom-ing injured; not digesting food properly and even indulging in too much sexual activity!

So, an ayurvedic practitioner's job is pretty complex, to put it mildly. However, ayurveda does produce remarkable results with even the tiniest adjustment: changing your diet or readjusting your working times can have surprising effects on your health. Even if you do decide that the complete ayurvedic package is too much to take en masse, it would still be well worth investigating some of its principles.

Ayurvedic philosophy is incredibly intricate and takes years of study to begin to comprehend. Put at its simplest, it teaches that each atom consists of five elements: its weight comes from earth, its cohesion from water, its energy from fire and its motion from air, while the space between its particles is composed of ether. Under this principle, the entire human body is composed of the five elements and it is thought that an excess of one or more elements can be the cause of imbalance and hence lead to illness.

The Doshas

Over the centuries, a kind of shorthand for working out imbalances evolved within ayurveda – the three *doshas*, or bioenergies, which are various combinations of the five elements. *Vata* is a combination of ether and air; *pitta* of fire with water; *kapha* of water and earth. In an ideal state, we would have all three doshas in perfect balance, but this is rare. Most of us have one or perhaps two which outweigh the others. The overall aim of ayurvedic medicine is to balance the doshas to restore health.

Your predominating dosha can be detected by a series of physical and emotional characteristics. For example, vata people are usually thin, agile, quick-thinking and restless; pitta people tend to be of medium build, competitive and make good leaders; kapha people are larger framed and are more placid in nature, possessing great reserves of strength and endurance. The aim of the practitioner is to coax all the elements into perfect balance so perfect health can follow. However complex the theory, the advice is very practical and down-to-earth. The ayurvedic practitioner seeks to balance the body, using primarily a combination of lifestyle advice, diet, exercise and herbal medicines. Massage, manipulation, marma therapy (similar to acupressure), neurotherapy, aromatherapy and sound therapy are also used. Yoga, meditation and deep breathing are highly recommended.

While all of these are gentle, non-invasive treatments, some ayurvedic physicians perform quite brutal techniques as well. The deep-cleansing process known as *panchakarma* can include therapeutic vomiting, enemas and purging. Nasal cleansing can be administered and, in cases of blood disorders, blood-letting is sometimes performed.

Ayurveda can be a tough therapy to take because, to achieve the best results, you do need to be totally dedicated to following the lifestyle and diet guidance. However, many Westerners are not willing to get up at 5 am, for example, or eat their main meal at lunchtime as advised. Practitioners and physicians vary in their insistence on rigidly following the rules: some are very dogmatic; others accept that ayurvedic routines can be difficult to adhere to in a Western lifestyle and more and more practitioners are adapting their cures for Western sensibilities. In addition, although ayurveda is considered an 'alternative' therapy, it can be (and often is) used alongside Western treatments.

There is little doubt that, in the hands of an experienced practitioner, ayurveda can achieve wonderful (some would say miraculous) results. At present, a number of research projects are being conducted to try to discover how these cures take place and to investigate the properties of several ayurvedic herbs and herbal preparations. Preliminary studies by the (American) National Cancer Institute research project indicate that a compound of herbs called *maharishi amrit kalash* has been found to possess anticarcinogenic and antineoplastic properties and a series of experiments carried out at South Dakota State University and the Ohio State University College of Medicine indicates that it 'may have great value in the prevention and treatment of cancer'.

How to find your Ayurvedic type

As we've already seen, we each contain within us the three doshas: *vata*, *pitta* and *kapha*. The dosha that dominates within our bodies gives rise to our prakruti, or body–mind type – the basic force that affects everything about us, from our shape and weight to our predisposition to different illnesses. Our *prakruti* will influence the kind of foods we should eat; the exercise we should take; even the kind of holiday we should enjoy.

Discovering your prakruti is really quite simple – just answer the questions opposite, ticking the answers which most apply to you.

Vata – air and space. Vata people eat little, usually preferring sweet, sour and salty foods, and they tend to be thin. Vatas are active, talkative and do not sleep much; their short-term memories are stronger than their long-term memories and they are often emotionally insecure. Vata elements are responsible for body motion, respiration, sensory impulses, autonomic mind function, circulation, separating digested from undigested food, regulation of menses and the passage of body fluids.

Pitta – fire. People dominated by the pitta element tend to become hot and sweaty easily, and have colour in their skin. They have strong appetites for spicy, sweet and bitter foods. Pittas are articulate and precise, and have strong memories; they can become fiercely angry and emotionally intense. The pitta element is responsible for vision, digestion, heat production, immunity, metabolism, the colour of the skin, organs and body fluids, appetite, thirst, suppleness and intellectual thought.

Kapha – earth and water. Kaphas tend to be large framed, stable and patient. They learn slowly, but have a good long-term memory. Kapha people sleep a lot and tend to be affectionate and emotionally secure. The kapha elements are responsible for maintaining the oiliness of the body and organs, general physical stability, virility, strength and the fluidity of muscular and joint movement.

YOUR BODY
1. What were you like as a child?
a) Small and thin
b) Average
c) Large and plump

2. What is your build now?
a) Thin build with light bones and prominent joints
b) Medium build and bone structure
c) Large-boned, quite heavy and dense in build

3. Do you put on weight?
a) Hardly ever
b) Both easily gain and easily lose weight
c) Find it hard to lose weight

4. What is your skin like?
a) Dry and delicate
b) Soft, maybe ruddy or freckled
c) Thick and oily

5. What kind of appetite do you have?
a) Irregular. You often snack or nibble, and can't finish a large meal
b) Good. You hate to skip meals and feel rotten if you do
c) Healthy. You like your food, but can miss meals without any ill effects

6. How do you walk?
a) Quickly, lightly – always in a hurry
b) Medium pace, determined and purposeful
c) Slowly, steadily and calmly

7. How do you sleep?
a) Lightly, with sleep often interrupted. You may suffer from insomnia
b) Regularly and soundly
c) Heavily and for a long time. You often oversleep or feel drowsy in the day

8. What kind of illnesses are you prone to?
a) Sharp pains, headaches, eczema, dry rashes, nervous disorders, gas or constipation
b) Rashes and allergies, inflammation, heartburn, ulcers, acidity, feverish complaints
c) Fluid retention, excess mucus, bronchitis, sinus problems, asthma, congestion

YOUR MIND AND EMOTIONS
1. What is your basic personality?
a) Enthusiastic, outgoing, talkative
b) Strong-minded and purposeful
c) Calm, placid and good-natured

2. What are you like at work?
a) Quick, imaginative and alert – you are a creative thinker. You hate rigid routine or discipline

b) Efficient, a natural leader. You like well-planned routines and tend to be a perfectionist
c) Calm and organized. You enjoy a regular routine and keep projects running along smoothly

3. How do you react to stress?
a) You become anxious and nervous
b) You become angry or irritable
c) You try to avoid it at all costs

4. How do you dream?
a) Frequently, but you often can't remember dreams on waking
b) Vividly, often in colour. You find it easy to remember your dreams
c) You only remember highly significant or clear dreams

5. How is your sex life?
a) It fluctuates – sometimes you love it, sometimes you aren't interested. You have an active fantasy life
b) Pretty average sex drive
c) You take a while to 'warm up', but then have intense sex – you love it and have great stamina

6. Do you save or spend money?
a) Spend it! You're an impulse buyer with a huge credit-card bill
b) Sensibly spend. You buy useful and classic items
c) Save. You always have enough money to get by

7. What is your memory like?
a) Quick to learn, quick to forget
b) Generally quite good
c) You take a while to learn, but your memory is excellent

8. How would you describe your lifestyle?
a) Erratic, always changing
b) Busy with plenty of plans – you achieve a lot
c) Steady and regular – you may feel rather stuck in a rut

ASSESSING YOUR SCORE

Simply add up the number of a's, b's and c's you have ticked. Predominantly a's means you are mostly a vata type; b's indicate pitta and c's indicate kapha. You may find two scores are equal or very close – it's common to be a combination. Some rare people possess all three doshas equally. Now turn the page to discover what your score means for your health and wellbeing.

What can Ayurveda help?

- Digestive problems such as stomach ulcers, chronic gastritis, acid indigestion, heartburn, constipation and flatulence benefit from ayurveda.
- Gynaecological problems such as menstrual and menopausal difficulties can be helped.
- Ayurveda helps with weight problems such as weight loss and weight gain.
- Skin complaints such as eczema, dermatitis, psoriasis and acne can be improved.

- Allergic conditions such as asthma, hayfever and sinus problems respond well.
- Problems with joints such as chronic pain, muscle tension, sciatica, rheumatism, arthritis and osteoporosis can be alleviated.
- It can help psychosomatic illnesses such as sleep disturbances, migraine and tension headaches, depression and anxiety attacks.
- Heart and blood-circulation problems such as angina, high blood pressure, palpitations and an irregular pulse can be treated.
- Some physicians have also treated conditions such as cancer, multiple sclerosis and myalgic encephalomyalitis (ME) with success – and there is research into HIV/AIDS.
- Ayurveda helps with addictions such as those to alcohol, smoking and drugs.

What can I expect from a session?

WHERE WILL I HAVE THE TREATMENT?
You will be lying on a special massage couch for massage and marma therapy. You will sit in a chair for consultations.

WILL I BE CLOTHED?
It depends. You will generally be completely naked for massage and fully clothed for other treatments.

WHAT HAPPENS?
A session will always begin with pulse diagnosis. The taking of pulses is an exact science – pulses are read in 12 positions. Practitioners will also want to know about your urine and stools, how you sleep, what you eat, how you think and feel. They will probably examine your eyes and your tongue, and they will also be watching how you talk and move.

After diagnosis comes treatment – and the range of treatments is vast. Without doubt, however, you will be given guidelines for healthy living and instructed in the diet that will soothe and counter imbalances in your body type. Ayurveda teaches that what is food for one person could be poison for another: your diet will be tailored precisely for your body type. Herbs are often prescribed. So, too, are yoga exercises and pranayama (breathing) exercises. If necessary, you will be prescribed marma therapy (see pages 18–20) or any one of the incredible range of massage therapies.

WILL IT HURT?
Marma therapy can be particularly painful. However, the other massage therapies don't generally hurt.

WILL ANYTHING STRANGE HAPPEN?
Ayurveda often feels very strange to Westerners. The massage therapies are quite unusual – you may find yourself being bathed in a continuous stream of warm oil, or having rings placed around your closed eyes while warm oil is poured over them. The enemas can take some getting used to as well.

WILL I BE GIVEN ANYTHING TO TAKE?
You may well be given herbal preparations. Your diet will often be modified or changed. Some practitioners recommend bastis (herbal enemas). And sometimes you might be asked to take ghee (clarified butter).

IS THERE ANY HOMEWORK?
Yes, there's plenty. Ayurveda teaches a whole system of lifestyle, so expect to be asked to adjust your eating, sleeping and working patterns; start or continue exercising; and perhaps to do yoga or breathing exercises as well.

Balancing the Doshas

Now you know which is your predominant dosha, you can learn how to balance it. Ayurveda is incredibly practical – there is not necessarily any need to take herbs or undergo complicated treatments; the first step is to make very simple changes in your everyday life.

Balancing Vata

- Above all else, you need regularity in your life. You will find this difficult, but do try because it will give you a far more steady and balanced output of energy. You will be able to keep going for far longer, rather than continue your usual pattern of expending masses of energy in short bursts, followed by periods of complete collapse.
- Make yourself eat your meals regularly, at the same time each day. Always sit down for your food – eating on the run or snatching snacks will aggravate vata very quickly.
- Try to go to bed at the same time each night and get up at the same time each morning. Going to bed early (about 10 pm is ideal) will make you less anxious and agitated.
- Learn to recognize when you are going into overdrive and consciously slow down. Meditation, yoga, chi kung or autogenic training could really help you.
- You love fast, high-energy sports and activities, but, to balance vata, you should try something more calming and lower in impact. Again yoga is great. So, too, is tai chi. If you always run or do high-impact aerobics, lessen the pace and try hill-walking or low-impact aerobics. Take a regular amount of steady exercise throughout the week, rather than doing nothing all week and then exhausting yourself with a two-hour squash marathon at the weekend.
- Try to avoid loud music, flashing lights and computer games. Calm, gentle, creative pursuits may sound boring to your swift brain, but taking up painting or tapestry could be just what you need. Cultivate the fine art of doing nothing.
- If you're going on holiday, resist the urge to book the 'learn a different sport each day' or 'seven locations in five days' type break. Instead, pick a beautiful spot and stay there. Give yourself sun, warmth and relaxation.
- Follow the vata-calming diet (see the guidelines on pages 15–16). Never eat very dry food, frozen foods or leftovers.
- Keep warm. Vata needs warmth in all senses – physical and spiritual. Place yourself in a safe, warm, caring environment. Saunas and steam rooms are wonderful for vata.
- Learn to express your feelings. Vatas often suppress their feelings, which aggravates their dosha.
- Get enough sleep. Vatas should avoid late nights and particularly shun jobs that involve night shifts.

Balancing Pitta

- Keep cool. Avoid extreme heat, stay out of very hot sun and keep clear of steam rooms and saunas (although you probably adore them). After a warm bath or shower, finish off with a cool rinse. Get out in the open air as much as you can, but, if it's hot, keep cool in the shade.
- You're normally highly organized, so introduce a little spontaneity into your life. Be careful you don't become too goal-oriented, too focused on objectives and nothing else. Try taking a walk 'just for the hell of it' or just sitting in the garden and gazing out of the window. Simply muse rather than doing something – very therapeutic for pitta.
- You will thrive on challenge, hate being bored and love competition. Obviously, it is important not to get bored, but don't take on too much or challenge yourself too far. Be very careful you don't end up sacrificing everything just to win.
- You can easily take sport too seriously and be far too competitive. Balance this by taking

up non-competitive activities as well, such as yoga, walking or Pilates. Do things for sheer fun. Water sports are calming and soothing for pitta and, of course, winter sports in the snow and ice will cool your fire.
- Pittas should watch their diet with great care (see the guidelines on page 16). Avoid, or at the very least cut right down on, oily and greasy foods, caffeine, salt, red meat, alcohol and highly spiced foods (things you will love).

Balancing Kapha

- Let go. Kaphas are great hoarders. You hold on to things – even weight, people and emotions. Loosen up and allow yourself to trust a little, to release anything you are holding on to too tightly. Trust there will always be enough.
- Allow change, unpredictability and excitement into your life. Kaphas love routine and feel safe and secure when everything stays the same, but taking the odd chance or allowing the pulse rate to speed up a little from time to time will give you a good energy boost.
- Vary the route you take to work; shift the furniture around in your office or home; if you always have a drink at 6 pm, go for a walk instead.
- Kaphas love to sit doing nothing in particular (Winnie the Pooh is a typical kapha!). To balance your dosha, you need to get your system moving, to give it a shake-up. Take on new activities and challenges that will stimulate you both physically and mentally. Try a new sport or night class, or see a different film to the kind you usually watch.
- Keep your activities varied: if you normally do aerobics, do step or circuits instead. Keep changing your routine in the gym or take a different route each time you jog.
- On holiday, kaphas are the ones whose idea of fun is flopping onto a sun lounger in the morning and being prized from it come dusk. To stimulate kapha, choose a touring holiday or an activity break.
- Follow the kapha diet on page 16. Avoid iced food and drinks; cut right down on sweet things and make sure you don't eat too much bread. Dairy produce will aggravate kapha – it produces mucus (a particular problem for the kapha type). Wheat can be a problem, too. Heavy, starchy foods are really unsuitable for kapha.

Ayurvedic eating

Food is medicine, according to ayurveda. If you eat the right foods, your body will automatically start to heal. Again, the philosophy is very complex, but, put simply, food possesses three basic qualities:

LIGHT (known as *satvic*): said to bring the psyche into a state of harmony. Foods with light qualities include vegetables and fruits, nuts, honey, milk and dairy produce, wheat, rice and rye. You should aim to make up most of your diet with foods with a light quality.

PASSIONATE (known as *rajastic*): said to stimulate the sensuality of the person, increasing motivation, ambition, jealousy, egotism. Foods with passionate qualities include all highly spiced, sour, salty, hot and dry foods, plus wine and beer, tea and coffee. You need a certain amount of these foods to sustain you in a tough world, but don't overdo them.

SLUGGISH (known as *tamasic*): foods with a sluggish quality increase pessimism, ignorance, greed, laziness, stinginess and feelings of inferiority. Some ayurvedic texts even go so far as to say they will seduce people into crime. Foods with a sluggish quality include all highly processed foods (canned, dried, frozen and 'quick' or convenience foods), peanuts, leftovers and overcooked food, strong alcoholic drinks and all meat and meat products. Naturally, it is advisable to avoid these as much as possible.

Food is also classified into six 'tastes' and six characteristics. The six tastes are: sweet, sour, salty, pungent (many spices and herbs come into this category), bitter (i.e. rhubarb, many greens) and astringent (certain vegetables and pulses).

The characteristics are: heavy or light (e.g. beef is heavy, while chicken is light; full-fat cheese is heavy, while low-fat cottage cheese is light); oily or dry (e.g. milk is oily, honey is dry); and hot or cold (in essence, rather than temperature – i.e. pepper is hot, while mint is cold). You should generally aim to include all of the six tastes in your diet, but avoid the characteristics that are known particularly to aggravate your predominating dosha (see the guidelines on pages 15–16).

The ten rules of healthy eating

1 Allow plenty of time to prepare and eat your food. Eat in a relaxed, congenial atmosphere and concentrate on what you're eating – don't read a book or watch television while having your meal. Always sit down to eat and take the time to savour your food.
2 The foods you eat should be attractive and wholesome – both to your taste buds and your eyes. Always prepare your table with care: use a fresh tablecloth and have fresh flowers or perhaps a candle as a centrepiece.
3 Try to eat at the same time each day. Be mindful of what you eat and be aware of your appetite – stop when you are not quite full. Never eat to excess. Eat your food slowly and chew each mouthful thoroughly, paying attention to the texture and taste of the food.
4 Always make sure you have digested your last meal before eating another. Generally, you should allow 3 to 6 hours between meals. Don't eat if you are not hungry.
5 Avoid ice-cold drinks – particularly around and with meals. Drink hot or warm water with your meals instead. If you want to eat or drink anything cold (such as ice cream), do so between meals – or warm your stomach with a cup of ginger tea beforehand, if you are having something cold.
6 Ideally, the bulk (if not all) of your diet should come from organic, locally produced, seasonal food. The majority of your meal should consist of warm, freshly prepared food, which is easier to digest.
7 Make lunch, the midday meal, the main meal of the day. Your digestion functions best between noon and 1 pm.
8 The digestive fire, known as *agni*, is low by evening, so make your evening meal small and easily digested. Avoid heavy dairy produce, animal protein and raw, cold foods at this time, as they are more difficult to digest.
9 Don't race off after your meal. Allow yourself a few minutes of calm relaxation. Relax, sit quietly and give thanks for your food. Take a gentle walk if you can, to aid digestion.
10 Notice how you feel after each meal. Become aware of what foods your body likes and doesn't like. What do certain foods do for your energy levels? Do any make your heart race or make you feel breathless, uncomfortable or bloated? Be guided by your body when it comes to your food choices.

Diet & the Doshas

Food is one of the prime ways we can balance the doshas. These are the foods that balance or soothe your main dosha.

FOODS TO SOOTHE VATA
People who are predominantly vata should ensure that, above all, they eat at regular times in a calm, relaxed atmosphere. Their diet should be warming and nourishing, with plenty of salty, sour and sweet tastes. So, boost the following in your diet:
• dairy produce – milk, cream, cheese, butter, yogurt, ghee (clarified butter)
• natural sweeteners – honey, cane sugar, maple syrup

- all types of nuts and seeds – but in small amounts
- chicken, duck, fish, turkey, seafood
- eggs
- sesame oil
- wheat and rice, cooked oats
- sweet, ripe fruits: bananas, apricots, mango, melon, papaya and peaches.
- vegetables cooked with a little added ghee: garlic and onions, asparagus, beetroot, carrots, cucumber, sweet potato, green beans. In moderation: potatoes, peas, spinach, courgettes (zucchini), tomatoes, celery.
- pulses (eat only in moderation): aduki beans (very occasionally), red lentils, black lentils (very occasionally), mung beans
- herbs: those with sweet and warming tastes such as basil, marjoram, coriander (cilantro), fennel, bay leaves, oregano, sage, tarragon, thyme
- spices: again, sweet and warming spices such as liquorice, mace, caraway, cardamom, cloves, cumin, cinnamon (shown opposite), ginger, mustard, black pepper, nutmeg (below)

FOODS TO SOOTHE PITTA

Pitta is hot and so pitta people need to cool themselves down. Anything that makes you hot – such as salt, hot and pungent spices and seasonings, and oil – should be avoided. Bitter and astringent tastes are useful for pitta. Pittas should aim for calm mealtimes, too – stress often causes them to miss meals or eat on the run.

These are the foods which particularly suit pittas:
- unsalted butter, ghee, milk, ice cream, cottage cheese
- almost all kinds of pulses and legumes, except for black and red lentils
- barley, cooked oats, wheat, white rice
- poultry, rabbit, fish (freshwater, in moderation)
- egg (but just the whites)
- all sweeteners except honey and molasses
- vegetables: asparagus, cucumber, broccoli, Brussels sprouts, cabbage, celery, green beans, all green leafy vegetables, mushrooms, potatoes, sweet peppers, courgettes (zucchini), bean sprouts, chicory
- ripe, sweet fruits: apples, coconut, figs, grapes, mangoes, cherries (but they must be sweet, rather than the sour varieties), raisins, prunes, lemons, oranges
- sunflower and pumpkin seeds
- coconut
- spices: cardamom, coriander (cilantro), cinnamon, saffron, ginger, turmeric, black pepper (in small amounts)
- herbs: dill, fennel, mint

FOODS TO SOOTHE KAPHA

Kapha people should aim for a light, dry, hot diet. Anything heavy, fatty or cold will weigh kapha down and make you sluggish and more prone than usual to putting on weight (a perennial kapha problem). Aim for low-fat, spicy, lightly cooked meals.

These foods will help balance your constitution if you are predominantly kapha:
- skimmed milk (or goat's milk), buttermilk, ghee (in small quantities only)
- all pulses except lentils, kidney beans and soya beans
- poultry, prawns (shrimp), game (in small, seasonal quantities only)
- sunflower and pumpkin seeds
- raw honey
- small amounts of oils and fat: ghee, almond oil, corn, sunflower oil
- barley, buckwheat, corn, maize, millet, rye, white rice (small quantities)
- most vegetables except cucumber, tomatoes, courgettes (zucchini), pumpkin, squash and olives

- fruit: apples, pears, pomegranates, cranberries, dates, figs, dried fruits
- herbs: all and plenty
- spices: all and plenty, especially ginger, coriander (cilantro), cloves, black pepper, turmeric, cardamom, cinnamon

Rules for a healthy lifestyle

- Get up between 4 am and 6 am! Ideally, you should have between 6 and 8 hours of sleep (but no more). Ayurveda teaches that the habit of going to bed late and sleeping in late can lead to all sorts of complaints, from digestive disorders to headaches and eye problems.
- Urinate first thing after rising. If it's difficult, drink a glass of water or herbal tea (not coffee). Next, attend to mouth hygiene: brush your teeth, clean your tongue and gargle with cold water. Rinse your eyes with cool water. Remember to trim fingernails and toenails every fifth day.
- Exercise. A long, fast walk, swimming or yoga is ideal.
- Massage after exercise reduces fat and removes dead skin. Rub oil into your entire body and then take a warm (body-temperature) bath to revitalize your body and stimulate your energy levels.
- As you leave the bath, dry and put on a little natural perfume. Dress in loose, comfortable, clean clothing.
- Take a few minutes for meditation, prayer or simply thinking about beautiful things.
- Then (at last) have breakfast. Breakfast should be eaten before 9 am. (No wonder you need an early start!)
- Lunch should be at least 3 hours later than breakfast – around 1 pm is fine. It should be the largest meal of the day, as this is when your body can most easily digest food.
- Dinner should be eaten no later than 9 pm – 6 pm is ideal. This meal should be quite light.
- You should aim to be in bed by 10 pm and asleep no later than 11 pm. If you are awake later, your body will move into a different dosha and you will find it even harder to fall asleep. Keep a window open in your bedroom – air should circulate freely. Sleep on the right side to promote digestion and have your head pointing either to the east or to the west. Do not share your room with animals.
- Sex is a strong part of ayurveda and is recommended in unrestricted amounts in winter. In spring and autumn, it is recommended no more than three times a week, while, in summer, according to the texts, you should only have sex two or three times a month.

Shirodhara

Shirodhara is one of a series of remarkable body treatments which form an essential part of ayurveda. It is an incredibly simple treatment: you lie down on a couch and a needle-thin stream of herbal oil, heated to a specific temperature, is poured continuously over the forehead. This usually lasts between half an hour and an hour, and is highly effective for balancing and settling vata disorders such as insomnia, anxiety and worry. It settles the mind and profoundly relaxes the central nervous system, giving the effect of a deep, silent meditative state. Best of all, shirodhara feels blissful.

There are a host of other ayurvedic massage techniques that might be prescribed for you:

Abhyanga

This is an incredibly relaxing massage which helps the body to release toxins. It is performed by two people working in perfect synchronization. There are three types of basic abhyanga, depending on your ayurvedic type – they vary in depth and speed of stroke, and in the type of oil used.

Vishesh

A firm, squeezing massage, designed to remove deep-rooted toxins, vishesh is quite a tough massage. It is particularly suitable for strong kapha people.

Garshan

This is a brisk, enlivening massage using raw silk gloves to create friction and static electricity on the surface of the skin. Garshan is very useful for weight loss.

Pizzichilli

This is known as the Royal Treatment and was once the preserve of Indian royalty. Literally gallons of warm oil are poured over the body, while two therapists gently massage in the oil. Pizzichilli relieves deep-seated aches and pains, and increases flexibility of the joints.

Marma Therapy

Anyone who wants to live long, appear young and remain in perfect health should look to their marmas. Here in the West, few people have even heard of the word marma, yet, to an Indian ayurvedic physician, the marmas are the key to health, emotional security, longevity and beauty – even life itself. The marmas are like the junction boxes of the body, 107 points or areas where nerves and muscles meet. While they stay uncongested, you will remain healthy and happy. If they become clogged or unbalanced, you could find your confidence failing alongside your health; both emotions and physiological functions become impaired if your marma points are out of alignment.

Ancient ayurvedic texts describe the marmas in precise detail. Centuries of observation had taught the ayurvedic surgeons that, if certain marmas were cut or damaged, death, disability, loss of function or pain would ensue.

Although they sound, at first hearing, very similar to the Chinese acupuncture points, the marmas differ in significant ways. They are connected directly with the nervous system, linking the body with the brain; they also lie deeper in the body than the acupuncture points and many cover an area of the body, rather than just a tiny point.

The reason why the marmas are so crucial is that they provide the links between body and mind. If the marma points are blocked, the nervous system cannot send clear messages to the brain. If there is a problem in the body, the alarm message sent from the body might simply not be able to get through. Not realizing anything is wrong, the brain would fail to mobilize the body's rescue forces to sort out the problem. The result would be that we fall ill.

Unfortunately, modern life is not easy on the marmas. We eat the wrong kind of diet, we don't exercise enough, we ingest and inhale vast quantities of pollutants and expose ourselves to a bombardment of stress almost every day of our lives. Although the marmas valiantly try to deal with the combined debris these abuses create, they often become overloaded and congested. It is easy to see why ayurvedic practitioners believe it is so important to keep your marmas in optimum condition for not only your physical, but also your emotional, wellbeing.

What can Marma Therapy help?

• Marma therapy can have a beneficial effect on a wide variety of conditions. It is ideal for

conditions which seem to have no physiological cause – vague aches and pains, and so-called psychosomatic conditions.
- It is deeply detoxifying and so therefore can help to treat conditions such as rheumatism and arthritis, weight problems, headaches and migraine.
- Patients report not just physiological improvements, but emotional benefits as well. Confidence is usually boosted. Anxiety, depression, fear and stress usually diminish.
- Marma therapy can be wonderful for low energy states and general weakness and fatigue.

What can I expect from a session?

WHERE WILL I HAVE THE SESSION?
You will be lying on a couch or on the floor.

WILL I BE CLOTHED?
Yes, you will remain fully clothed.

WHAT HAPPENS?
Marma therapy works by the therapist manually stimulating the marma points with either direct pressure or insistent massage. Before treatment, the practitioner will take your pulses and ask to see your tongue. You will then be asked to lie down on the couch or floor.

Marma therapy is certainly no feel-good massage: some points are very tender and the touch is very hard. You may also find the practitioner shaking your limbs or giving a sharp slap to the soles of the feet. Sometimes, he or she will measure your limbs to check on imbalances.

For the final stage of the treatment, a light oil may be used to rub up and down either side of the spine.

WILL IT HURT?
Yes, quite possibly. Some people may even find the touch too harsh to tolerate.

WILL ANYTHING STRANGE HAPPEN?
You may feel the blockages as the practitioner works on them – like bubbles under the skin.

WILL I BE GIVEN ANYTHING TO TAKE?
No, medication is not part of the treatment.

IS THERE ANY HOMEWORK?
Yes, you may well be given adjustments to make in your lifestyle and particularly in your diet.

Tuning up the Marmas – home techniques

Fortunately, there are plenty of simple do-it-yourself techniques for keeping your marmas clear which you can practise without the aid of a therapist.
- The marmas can be activated and toned through yoga. Try to practise at least a few yoga postures every day – they stretch the marma points. The Salutation to the Sun series of postures is an ideal toning routine for the marmas. Gentle exercise such as walking and swimming can help, too.
- A cluster of important marma points can be found on the soles of the feet. Giving your feet a gentle foot massage with sesame oil for 3 to 5 minutes a day will be highly beneficial. If you do this just before bedtime, it will soothe the nervous system and help you get a restful night's sleep. Allow your bowl of sesame oil to sit on a radiator or in

a *bain-marie* for a while to warm. Take your time and slowly massage each part of the foot with a gentle, circular motion.
- There are three major marma points which should be gently massaged every day. Use a light, circular motion, taking a few minutes at each site.

    There is a head marma situated between the eyebrows, extending to the centre of the forehead. Gently massaging this area while your eyes are closed is good for relieving anxiety, headaches and mental strain. It will also help you to sleep well at night.

    The heart marma is located just below the sternum, where the rib cage ends, and massaging the heart marma will help settle upset emotions.

    Massaging the marma point on the lower abdomen, about 10 cm (4 in) below the navel, will help the intestinal tract and ease constipation and gas.
- Make sure your diet is as good as possible (see the guide to ayurvedic eating on pages 14–16). If possible, choose organic wholefoods low in acid and avoid processed or highly refined foods, all of which can clog the marmas. In addition, all meals should be eaten slowly and calmly at regular times: snacking between meals is forbidden, as the food will not digest properly and waste will be dumped at the marma points.

Neurotherapy

Practitioners of neurotherapy believe they can cure most of our problems by walking all over us – literally. In India, where the therapy originated, film stars, politicians and government ministers are ignoring orthodox Western medicine in favour of neurotherapy, drawn by tales of amazing cures. It may sound bizarre, but the entire therapy has been very precisely analysed and researched; it is based on a deep understanding of physiology and anatomy.

Unlike many alternative traditions, neurotherapy is refreshingly down-to-earth. Although their field is rooted in the ancient system of ayurveda, neurotherapists tend to talk in language that any medical doctor would recognize and understand, and even use themselves: of hormones and enzymes; blood cholesterol levels and peptides; glands and nerve reflexes. Neurotherapy acts through the body's nadis or nerve channels directly on the organs and glands, fine-tuning the biochemical balance of the body.

Therapists don't seek a quick fix; they are like genealogists of the body, not content until they have ferreted back to the great-great-grandparent of your symptoms. Take the case of rheumatoid arthritis, for example. This causes the joints to become inflamed and eventually degenerate because of an accumulation of poisonous acids in them. The root cause, however, may well lie further afield: the pancreas might not be producing sufficient alkaline salts to neutralize the acidic foods coming from the stomach, for instance. The intestines cannot then properly digest the food and the excretory system cannot properly get rid of the acids. The subsequent malfunctioning of the endocrine glands can then cause problems in the auto-immune system.

While Western doctors would tend to prescribe drugs to ease the symptoms, neurotherapists assert that, instead of giving the body synthetic medicine, they can stimulate the body to produce the biochemicals it needs by itself.

This is where the feet come in. Pressure is placed on various parts of the body (either the organ or gland itself, or on the connecting nerves), using the insteps of the feet to provide a kind of suction effect. Rhythmic pressure on the precise spot will apparently stimulate the ailing organ or underproductive gland.

What can neurotherapy help?

- Digestive disorders (irritable bowel syndrome, gastritis, gallstones, colitis etc.) can be alleviated.
- Back problems (injuries, spondilytis etc.) respond well.

- It is good for hormonal imbalances (such as premenstrual syndrome, menopausal problems, thyroid problems and pituitary malfunctioning).
- Some people have found neurotherapy very helpful following a stroke and it has also had beneficial effects on multiple sclerosis, arthritis, cerebral palsy and Down's syndrome.
- Enthusiasts have found they have lost weight and conquered insomnia. They even say it can cure psychiatric illness.
- Some people should avoid neurotherapy: it cannot be used on hernias (other than hiatus hernias); people with pacemakers cannot be treated; and nor can it be used if someone has undergone a hip replacement.

What can I expect from a session?

WHERE WILL I HAVE THE TREATMENT?
You will be lying on the floor between two chairs.

WILL I BE CLOTHED?
Yes, you remain fully clothed throughout.

WHAT HAPPENS?
Neurotherapy sessions are surprisingly short and sweet. In India, practitioners can treat up to 90 patients in one day. In the West, the initial consultation takes an hour with follow-up treatments lasting just 30 minutes. The first appointment is taken up almost entirely with completing a detailed questionnaire. In particular, the therapist needs to know about any drugs that are being taken; as neurotherapy works directly on the glands, its results are often instantaneous and powerful.

You will then be asked to lie down, fully clothed, on a thick towel on the floor, with a rolled-up towel positioned under your knees for support.

Two chairs are placed on either side of your body, close to your hips. The practitioner then feels your abdomen, pressing firmly under the ribcage. This process (known as *nabi diagnosis*, similar to the hara diagnosis used in shiatsu) has been practised in India for thousands of years and is held to be highly precise. Balancing his or her weight on the chairs, the therapist places his or her feet on the inside of your thighs and gently rocks from side to side. This process is then repeated several times before you are asked to get up.

WILL IT HURT?
No. Surprisingly, neurotherapy is not at all painful.

WILL ANYTHING STRANGE HAPPEN?
Within minutes, you may well notice changes such as tenderness in the lymph glands.

WILL I BE GIVEN ANYTHING TO TAKE?
Neurotherapy does not use herbs or supplements, but neurotherapists will often recommend particular diets or certain foods to help heal conditions.

IS THERE ANY HOMEWORK?
Although the results can be swift and strong, you are still expected to put in some hard work towards leading a healthier life. Imbalances in the endocrine system most frequently occur because of the way we live and our bad habits. As a result, practitioners frequently teach patients how to breathe fully and properly, and will often demand dietary changes.

2 Chinese Medicine

In the old days in China, you paid your doctor while you were well and stopped paying him when you fell ill. Can you imagine a modern Western physician daring to launch such a scheme? Practitioners of traditional Chinese medicine had no such fears: their system of preventative medicine worked superlatively.

Patients were taught a combination of good diet, good exercise and good breathing technique. If a patient *did* fall sick, there were powerful ways to bring him or her back to health: acupuncture, herbalism and massage. Sickness was simply not a way of life – surely a tempting enough reason to investigate this incredible holistic system of healing.

Nowadays, in the West, we generally use only a small part of traditional Chinese medicine. Many people practise solely acupuncture; others purely herbalism. Both can have powerful effects on their own, but, if you really want to use this therapy in its most potent form, seek out a practitioner who can counsel you on all aspects of the Chinese way to health. Once you are eating, exercising and breathing properly, you shouldn't need more than a quarterly check-up and perhaps the odd tweak of a needle or the stray tonic to keep you in perfect health.

From the earliest times, people have stumbled across the healing powers of certain foods and herbs. But how did they discover that sticking a needle in a certain part of the body could have an effect on other parts, even curing disease? Some people say that acupuncture developed out of marma therapy (see ayurveda, pages 18–20). Others think that, after battles, the Chinese noticed some curious side effects of arrow wounds. If the victim survived his wound, sometimes he would discover that a formerly chronic disease had mysteriously improved, or even vanished. From these observations, they surmise, acupuncture was developed.

The underlying philosophy behind traditional Chinese medicine is that good health revolves around the correct flow of *qi*, or *chi*, the subtle energy of the body. Qi flows around the body in channels called *meridians*, and along the meridians lie hundreds of points which link the various organs and functions of the body. While Western doctors often scorn this idea, new instruments such as the PIP scanner (see electrocrystal therapy on pages 135–6) have actually confirmed what the Chinese have known for years: the position of the meridians and the acupuncture points.

If we look after ourselves, eat the right kinds of foods and undertake the right kinds of exercise, we can increase the amount of qi in our bodies. If we fall into bad ways, our levels of qi drop or are blocked and the consequence is lack of vital energy, emotional distress or even disease. The entire Chinese life view is immensely complex and, some might say, almost obsessive. Qi can be depleted or lost through too much, too little or the wrong kind of food, drink, exercise, work and even sex. Even your emotions can fall out of balance and affect your health.

Yin & Yang

According to traditional Chinese medicine, the world can be divided into two forces, *yin* and *yang*. Yin is considered to be dark, cold, negative, passive and feminine, while yang is light, warm, positive, active and male. Disturb the balance of yin and yang, and the result is disharmony, possibly ill health. In addition, there are the five elements to consider. Every one of us contains the elements of fire, earth, air (known as metal), water and wood. When a traditional Chinese medicine practitioner diagnoses, he or she does not just check for the flow of qi, but also looks to see how much of each element is within the body and what kind of energy is being transmitted. It is then possible to stimulate or quieten unbalanced organs or body systems through food, exercise, massage, herbs or the needles of acupuncture.

What can traditional chinese medicine help?

- Almost every condition will respond well to traditional Chinese medicine.
- Chinese herbs have become famous for treating eczema and other skin conditions.
- Acupuncture is well known as an aid to dieting and giving up smoking.
- Acupuncture also has good effects on emotional and psychological problems.
- A huge variety of conditions respond well to acupuncture – from acute problems such as headaches, coughs and colds to long-standing chronic conditions such as angina, irritable bowel syndrome, premenstrual syndrome, rheumatism and eczema.
- It can help relieve pain and has even been used with great success in childbirth.
- Some practitioners report good results with infertility.

What can I expect from a session?

WHERE WILL I HAVE THE TREATMENT?
You will be sitting in a chair for the initial diagnosis and lifestyle counselling. Acupuncture and tuina are carried out while you are lying on a couch.

WILL I BE CLOTHED?
You will be asked to remove some clothing for acupuncture. Otherwise, you will be fully clothed.

WHAT HAPPENS?
You will be asked a few questions about your health and past medical history; however, most traditional Chinese medicine practitioners can tell exactly what is going on in your body by taking your pulses and looking at your face, eyes and tongue.

If you are having acupuncture, you will be asked to lie down on a couch. Many acupuncturists use moxa, a herbal mixture which is placed on the acupoint and set alight. When it becomes warm, you tell the practitioner and it is whisked away before it burns the skin. The needle is then inserted and either left there or twisted in and then pulled out directly. This process will continue on a variety of points; some are in very strange places (such as the palate and the pubis!).

If you have a herbal consultation, you will be given a precise mixture of herbs to take – either in pill form or, more likely, loose to be brewed as a tea.

WILL IT HURT?
Acupuncture can be slightly painful, depending on the practitioner and the technique used. If needles are inserted superficially, it doesn't hurt at all. Sometimes, however, they may be inserted deeply and twisted, which can be a somewhat uncomfortable sensation. If tuina massage (see below) is part of your treatment, it can at times be very deep and strong.

WILL ANYTHING STRANGE HAPPEN?

You may feel a tingling or surge of released energy when a needle is inserted. Some people find that old emotions are released through acupuncture or tuina (see below). Also, Chinese herbs can have very swift reactions – you may find a cold, for example, clears almost instantly once you begin herbal treatment, or that you experience a sudden rush of energy.

WILL I BE GIVEN ANYTHING TO TAKE?

Yes, herbal preparations are often included in traditional Chinese medicine. These can be in pill or dried form. If taken in tea form (which is common), some of these taste quite unpleasant. You may also be asked to alter your diet.

IS THERE ANY HOMEWORK?

Yes. Most probably, you will be asked to practise good breathing techniques and to make lifestyle changes. Some practitioners may suggest that you take up chi kung or tai chi.

Tuina

Tuina gives a wake-up call to the whole body. It's an exciting and energizing system of massage that leaves your body feeling as if it has been given a thorough spring clean. Its effects on the mind are equally uplifting. Yet tuina is virtually unknown and unused here in the West.

In China, however, the story is totally different. There, it is as well established and respected as acupuncture and Chinese herbal medicine. Tuina massage is routinely used in Chinese hospitals – primarily to treat pain, but also in the treatment of many common ailments. The words *tui* and *na* literally mean 'push' and 'grasp'. This profound, invigorating and energizing form of massage and manipulation focuses deep pressure along the energy lines (known as meridians) and acupuncture points of the body. Tuina's aim is to release blocked energy and restore a balanced flow throughout the entire body, promoting a wondrous sense of health and vitality.

What can tuina help?

- Tuina is superlative for treating neck, shoulder and back pain, sciatica, frozen shoulders, tennis elbow and migraines.
- It can produce profound shifts in emotional wellbeing and is wonderful for beating stress.
- Many conditions can respond well to tuina – including digestive problems, menstrual irregularities and respiratory ailments.

What can I expect from a session?

WHERE WILL I HAVE THE TREATMENT?

You will be sitting in a chair and/or lying on the floor or a couch.

WILL I BE CLOTHED?

Yes, you are usually treated with all your clothes on.

WHAT HAPPENS?

Before the treatment, the therapist will ask a few questions about your health; whether you have had any injuries or serious illnesses, or if you are pregnant. Tuina is not suitable for people with fragile bones or osteoporosis, and practitioners also need to be very careful in treating those with cancer or heart problems. Certain points are avoided in pregnancy because they could induce labour. You are then asked to sit upright in a chair. The name *tuina* may mean to push and grasp, but your body will also be shaken, squeezed, pulled, rotated, rocked and rolled! At times, it feels like the deep-tissue work of Rolfing and Hellerwork (see pages 104–6, at others like osteopathic manipulation. The treatment starts with your neck and shoulders, before moving down your arms.

You will then move onto a couch and your back, buttocks and thighs will be pounded and kneaded. Finally, you are asked to sit on the floor with your legs stretched out in front. There is a pressure on your spine and, before you realize what is happening, your vertebrae 'pop' in swift succession like a strip of bubblewrap.

WILL IT HURT?
The tuina touch is very deep and can be painful. If you like to doze off during a massage or have a very low pain threshold, this really isn't for you.

WILL ANYTHING STRANGE HAPPEN?
As with most forms of bodywork, you may experience old memories resurfacing.

WILL I BE GIVEN ANYTHING TO TAKE?
No, medication is not part of the treatment

IS THERE ANY HOMEWORK?
You may be given moves to practise on yourself at home, or asked to make adjustments to your diet or lifestyle.

Home Tuina session

Note: This tuina massage is generally suitable for everyone, but do not massage on inflamed or broken skin, or over skin conditions such as eczema, psoriasis or shingles. You should also not use this massage on anyone with osteoporosis (brittle bones).

1 Your partner should be seated in a comfortable, upright chair with good back support, hands resting in the lap, feet firmly placed on the floor. Standing behind your partner, stroke lightly along the tops of the shoulders. Then squeeze gently along each shoulder with the whole hand, gradually increasing the pressure and starting to knead with the heel of the hand. As you feel your partner begin to relax, knead with the thumb, feeling for any tender or knotted tissue. Grasp the top of the shoulder and squeeze the large muscle there deeply, giving it a slight shake. To achieve the best results, spend at least 10 minutes on this step. These techniques unblock the energy channels from the head to the shoulders, significantly raising your energy levels.

2 Using your thumb and first two fingers, squeeze the muscles on either side of the neck vertebrae while the other hand lightly supports the forehead. Progress from light to strong pressure, with a definite kneading action. Work from the base of the neck up to the region just beneath the skull, lifting the hand between each position. Change hands frequently. Spend at least 5 minutes on this step. This technique stimulates the bladder and gall bladder meridians, sweeping away the tension that leads to headaches and relieving stiff and aching neck muscles.

3 Standing to the right-hand side of your partner's chair, put your right foot on the chair so your thigh is about level with his or her armpit. With your left hand, grasp his or her right wrist and raise the arm so it rests gently across your knee. Turn the wrist away from you. Grasping the muscle on the top of the shoulder with your right hand, squeeze firmly and knead deeply between your fingers and the heel of your hand. Continue like this down the arm. Repeat several times, then squeeze with the fingers and thumb lightly all the way down the arm, giving a slight lift between each position. Change hands frequently. Squeezing and kneading clears the energy channels in the shoulders, loosening the muscles.

4 Support your partner's right arm between your hands, just below the armpit. The arm should be completely relaxed. Using the palms in opposition technique (one palm moves in the opposite direction to the other), rub rapidly to and fro, massaging the arm muscles down to the wrist. This technique powerfully stimulates the flow of energy in all the meridians of the arm, which particularly helps the small intestines regain balance.

5 Hold your partner's right hand firmly with both hands, your thumbs together at the top of the wrist. Raise the arm to just below the horizontal and pull gently to loosen the shoulder joint. Then shake 20–30 times with small up-and-down movements. This technique greatly relieves shoulder stiffness, as well as pain in the arm and shoulder area, and the side of the neck. When the correct energy balance is established in your neck, shoulders and arms, you can feel like a new person.

6 Repeat steps 3, 4 and 5 on the left shoulder and arm. You should aim to spend about 10 minutes altogether on steps 3, 4 and 5 on each arm.

Good healthkeeping – the Chinese way

There are simple changes we can all make to our daily lives which can help us to live healthier, and even longer, lives.

A good diet is crucial. The first rule is to eat sparingly. The Chinese say you should eat until you are 70–80 per cent full. All food should be chewed thoroughly to allow the enzymes in the saliva to start digestion. Liquids should also be sipped, rather than gulped.

Avoid extremes of temperature – the Chinese tend not to eat or drink things that are either very hot or very cold. Ideally, food should be steamed, poached or stir-fried.

The traditional Chinese diet follows the World Health Organization guidelines almost exactly (see page 57), being high in complex carbohydrates, vegetables and fruits, while low in saturated fat. Fish is rated highly and meat is eaten only in small quantities. Chinese physicians have always recommended eating 'earth' chickens, or free-range chickens, as we know them.

The Chinese diet avoids dairy produce, as it is believed to cause allergies and infections. Eggs are eaten only rarely. The Chinese also avoid most of the nightshade family of vegetables, which includes potatoes, tomatoes and peppers (interestingly, modern nutritionists find that these foods can cause problems for quite a few people). Caffeine and tobacco should also be shunned.

Grains are rated very highly, with rice considered to be the most nourishing of all grains. Pulses such as lentils, aduki beans, kidney beans, chickpeas, mung beans and tofu (made from soya beans) are also important mainstays of the Chinese diet.

Vegetables are usually cooked, as they are considered much easier for the body to assimilate in that form. Also, cooked vegetables are believed to build up the body, while cold vegetables have a more eliminating action.

Red meat is very rarely eaten and then only when the body is depleted – it is considered very rich and to cause aggression and irritability in large doses. However, it can be therapeutic – e.g. a woman might eat a nourishing lamb stew after her period to regain blood and energy.

The chinese kitchen medicine cabinet

Sun Ssu-mo, an ancient Chinese physician in the Tang Dynasty, correctly diagnosed and cured beriberi, the nutritional deficiency disease caused by a lack of thiamine (vitamin B1) – 1,000 years before European doctors. He wrote: 'A truly good physician first finds out the cause of the illness and, having found that, he first tries to cure it with food. Only when food fails does he prescribe medication.'

Barley meal helps the digestion and drains what the Chinese call 'damp heat' – moving away foods that are stagnant in the system. Boil with rice for two hours.

Brussels sprouts are rich in alkalizing elements when lightly steamed, and particularly good for the pancreas.

Cherries are detoxifying, work as a laxative and stimulate the nervous system. The darker the cherries, the more therapeutic their value.

Chicken raises qi (energy) and is generally uplifting.

Cinnamon bark and euconia bark both possess aphrodisiac qualities.

Cucumber is rich in potassium, sodium and phosphorus. It is good for the nails and hair, as well as promoting excretion of waste through the kidneys.

Ginseng is an energy tonic to lift spirits and raise energy. It is very useful for those who are run down after an illness. Ginseng is also good for mental and physical stamina. (Note: contraindicated for high blood pressure, severe headaches or fever.)

Grapes are often used to cure constipation and gastritis, and as general detoxifiers. They also alkalize the digestive tract and bloodstream. Dark grapes are best.

Horseradish and lemon juice provides quick relief from mucus congestion – useful for coughs, colds, flu, asthma and pneumonia.

Lycii berries tonify the blood. Put them in buns or sprinkle them on porridge.

Mushrooms Shiitake mushrooms are often used as energy raisers. Rei-gen mushrooms are used as immune stimulants said to raise the white blood cell count. Often used by those with HIV/AIDS, they can also be used by anyone for their calming effects. They are said to alleviate stress and help you work with more vision.

Raw beetroot juice is a natural kidney cleanser, dissolving and eliminating any gravel.

Raw carrot and spinach juice detoxifies the digestive tract and helps normal bowel function. It is also used for tonsillitis and pneumonia, can help with rheumatism and colitis, and is believed to strengthen the heart and ease menstrual problems.

Raw, crushed garlic (above left) contains allicin, a powerful natural antibiotic and fungicide that helps prevents colds and flu, and is said to raise libido.

Raw tomato (left) is believed to reduce inflammation of the liver.

Red meat is helpful for blood. It is eaten very rarely by the Chinese, but some practitioners recommend women eat red meat after their periods to make new blood. A typical recipe is to cook lamb with Chinese angelica and lycii berries.

Schizandra helps focus the mind and is useful for those who are studying.

3 The Ancient Wisdom of Other Cultures

Ayurveda and traditional Chinese medicine are the best-known ancient systems of holistic healthcare, but there are many others. Some have been lost to us over the centuries because their wisdom was not written down and the oral tradition has dwindled in recent times. Others are still used and are gradually becoming better known in the West. Over the next few pages, we'll look at three fascinating systems.

Mongolian Healing

Could you blame your illness on your past lives? Maybe you are under the weather because your stars are unfavourable this year? Or perhaps you are being blighted by an evil spirit? Mongolian medicine goes way beyond the merely mechanical – it is based on the belief that health is a fusion of physical, psychological and spiritual. Prayers are as likely to be offered as pills, and exorcisms performed alongside acupuncture. It may sound bizarre, but the latest psychoneurimmunology (the science of mind–body medicine) research would probably agree with many of Mongolian healing's precepts. It also predates the concepts of quantum physics by several millennia, insisting that time is relative (the past and future affect the present) and that we are not separate from our surroundings.

Mongolian medicine was ancient when Genghis Khan rampaged across Central Asia with his hordes. At its heart is what is known as *em-dom*, an ancient folk medicine which has been retained in its purity and offers some unusual (to put it mildly) remedies. Horse milk is used to treat lung complaints. An infection in the umbilical cord of a newborn is cured by burning a piece of the mother's hair, grinding it into ash and putting it on the sore place – it is said to heal overnight. There are incredibly arcane formulae for everything from soothing mouth ulcers to promoting youthfulness.

Mongolian medicine is said to be as ancient as the great healing systems of China, Tibet, the Middle East (tibb) and India (ayurveda), if not more so. In fact, it shares many techniques with them – the use of herbs, moxibustion (the burning of herbs on the skin), acupuncture, massage and manipulation techniques. Even its spiritual practices are not dissimilar – although this side of traditional Eastern medicine is generally played down in the West.

What can Mongolian Healing help?

- Mongolian physicians will treat almost anything.
- Digestive and hormonal problems appear to respond well.
- It is said to improve longevity and make you feel more youthful.
- Mongolian massage is highly effective for back pain, stress-related problems and digestive troubles, and it is claimed that it can even help cellulite.
- It is said to heal psychic wounds and is ideal for people who want greater self-awareness.

What can I expect from a session?

WHERE WILL I HAVE THE TREATMENT?
You will be sitting in a chair for the consultation. If you need massage or acupuncture, you will lie on a couch.

WILL I BE CLOTHED?
You will be fully clothed for the consultation, but down to only underwear for chua ka, the massage.

WHAT HAPPENS?
Diagnosis is swift and efficient. As with ayurveda and traditional Chinese medicine, the practitioner will read your pulses, check your tongue and scrutinize your face. You will then be given a prescription to take. It's a very quick, down-to-earth session. Mongolian massage, chua ka, has been described as 'reflexology for the body' and it feels as if every acupressure point is being hit in turn. It's a really deep, powerful and satisfying massage.

WILL IT HURT?
Acupuncture can be uncomfortable and the massage can be very strong. At times it is almost painful, but the pain is forgotten as your body releases its tension – it's that weird kind of 'good hurt'.

WILL ANYTHING STRANGE HAPPEN?
You will be checked for evil spirits! The physician may decide you need a ceremony or ritual to help your problem.

WILL I BE GIVEN ANYTHING TO TAKE?
Yes, you may be given powders to dissolve in water, or pills.

IS THERE ANY HOMEWORK?
You may be asked to make some adjustments to your lifestyle.

Tibb or Unani medicine

Tibb is a hidden treasure in the world of natural health. A holistic system of medicine, tibb has been practised across vast areas of the world (Persia and Turkey, in particular) for thousands of years. Even today, it is still the main source of medicine in large areas of India, Pakistan, Bangladesh, Afghanistan, Malaysia and the Middle East. Practitioners say it incorporates knowledge from ancient Egyptian and Greek medicine, from the Chinese and Indian traditions, and from the ancient healing wisdom of Persia and the Middle East. Its extensive pharmacopoeia of herbs is now being investigated by Western pharmaceutical companies in the belief that tibb could hold the secrets to cures for many modern illnesses.

At first sight, tibb (which is also known as unani medicine, Sufi medicine or Graeco-Arabic medicine) appears little different from traditional Chinese or ayurvedic medicine. Like these, tibb recognizes vital energy (known in Arabic as *qawa*); it shares the concept that medicine needs to be holistic, to look at the whole person; it regards the correct balance of elements within the body as essential to health; and it uses a battery of herbal remedies to combat modern ills. However, although the basic philosophy of tibb shares much with its ancient cousins, it has unique strengths and qualities that make it worthy of a wider recognition around the world.

First, tibb is a very gentle medicine. Where Chinese doctors would treat first with diet, tibb physicians will look at lifestyle. They start at the most subtle levels, trying to adjust a person's breathing. It's a small change, but it can have a huge effect. Next, they attend to the emotions. In India, Pakistan and Bangladesh, where tibb is taught in universities, a major part of the hakim or practitioner's training involves counselling and psychotherapy. Tibb teaches that what a person thinks and imagines can affect his or her health profoundly.

Next, they investigate sleep and sleeping patterns, eating patterns and bowel movement. They will study your working life and how you relax, and try to find ways of making your life work for you in the most healthy yet realistic ways. Then, and only then, would they use herbs if necessary. If you had a structural problem, they might employ osteopathic manipulations or massage techniques (or refer you to other practitioners). Finally, if they felt your problem had a deeper, spiritual basis, they would use what is known as *logotherapy*, finding ways that fit your belief system or religion to soothe your very soul. So, tibb is holistic in the true sense of the word – the physician is looking at every patient on four levels: the physical, the emotional, the intellectual and the spiritual, and treating accordingly.

What can Tibb help?

- Tibb has good results with all manner of problems, both acute and chronic. Physicians say there are few conditions tibb ultimately cannot help – although they won't deal with accident or emergency cases.
- It is excellent if your problem has a psychological or spiritual aspect.
- It has good results for a variety of skin disorders and for respiratory conditions.
- In tibb, there is a large variety of herbal tonics that regulate and boost energy. There is even a hoard of supposedly highly potent aphrodisiacs.
- It often helps conditions which have proved resistant to other therapies.

What can I expect from a session?

WHERE WILL I HAVE THE TREATMENT?
You will be sitting in a comfortable chair for the consultation.

WILL I BE CLOTHED
Yes, you will be fully clothed.

WHAT HAPPENS?
The hakim starts with simple questions on your health and lifestyle. He will be keen to know about your birth. (For example, was it difficult? Tibb recognizes many problems as arising from traumatic births.) He will ask about your work, about your eating and exercising habits, your sleep and ways of relaxing. He will also want to know whether you have had any accidents or serious illnesses. It is like talking to a doctor and psychotherapist rolled into one – a wonderful combination. Then your wrist is taken to read your pulses. The hakim will also be assessing your body shape, complexion and whole manner for clues to your basic constitution or *mijaz*. In addition, he will look at your tongue and minutely observe your irises.

You will then be given your prescription, which might include some pampering sessions, gardening for earthing your energy, or perhaps some time out and relaxation, alongside medication.

WILL IT HURT?
No, this is not a painful therapy.

WILL ANYTHING STRANGE HAPPEN?
Some people may find the emphasis on spiritual and psychic matters unusual and perhaps a little disturbing.

WILL I BE GIVEN ANYTHING TO TAKE?

Yes, you may be given some tiny pills to take.

IS THERE ANY HOMEWORK?

Yes, you will be expected to make adjustments in your lifestyle.

Tibb home help

- Get up early – ideally, before sunrise and certainly before 7 am. Drink a little warm water and honey on rising to prevent constipation.
- Always eat a good breakfast. Skimping on breakfast or avoiding it altogether will lower your energy levels. Lunch should be a reasonable size, while the evening meal should be light and eaten at least two hours before bedtime. This regime should also regulate your weight – tibb teaches that most Western obesity is caused by eating too much too late at night and not enough at breakfast.
- Tibb emphasizes regular exercise to keep you healthy in body and mind. Walking is excellent.
- Make sure you get enough relaxation. Too many people in the West today are over-stimulated. If you always feel tired, on a day off, take half an hour's siesta in the afternoon. Have a warm bath with essential oils (lavender is excellent). Massage your feet or head with light oils.
- Incorporate spirituality into your life. Whether it involves prayer, meditation or simple contemplation of the beauty in the world, just ten minutes a day will help bring you peace.
- Don't go to bed too late. Our natural clock would take us to bed no more than a couple of hours after sunset. Try to be in bed by at least 11 pm.
- Cultivate good sleep. If you have trouble sleeping, try meditating before sleep or experiment with gentle massage – on your feet or head. A warm, milky drink is comforting. Start by sleeping on your right side – this promotes restful sleep.

Tibetan medicine

Tibetan medicine is ancient and venerable. It also appears to work – startlingly well. Reports have suggested that Tibetan physicians have cured 'incurable' diseases and many desperate people have flown thousands of miles to ask their opinions and to take their unique herbal preparations known as 'precious pills'. The Tibetan tradition of healing has always remained rather arcane and unapproachable simply because few Westerners had the basic tools (a working knowledge of modern and ancient Tibetan) to learn the system, or the patience to complete the training (it takes at least 10 years).

It can be hard to find a bona fide Tibetan physician in the West. However, increasing numbers of Westerners are taking up the knowledge and many are offering a combination of Tibetan massage and nutritional and lifestyle counselling.

Tibetans classify all of life into five energies which combine to create three 'humors' – air, bile and phlegm. Air controls breathing, speech and muscular activity, the nervous system, thought processes and your emotional attitude. Bile governs heat in the body, the liver and the digestive tract. Phlegm controls the amount of mucus in the body and also regulates the immune system. When all the humors are in balance within your body, you will enjoy perfect health. When one or more becomes aggravated or sluggish, problems will occur.

It sounds simple, but Tibetan healing is so precise and so complex that it can be mind-boggling: it takes a very experienced physician to bring about the kind of 'miracle' cures that occur. However, with just a little knowledge we could all make ourselves healthier.

Diet is very important and practitioners believe that often food is the only medicine required to obtain the necessary balance for good health and wellbeing.

What can Tibetan healing help?

- Tibetan medicine can benefit most conditions, particularly if you see a fully qualified physician.
- The massage is deeply stress-relieving and can help a wide variety of stress-related disorders.
- You should become more balanced, in both mind and body.
- Digestive problems and hormonal problems seem to respond well to Tibetan medicine.

What can I expect from a session?

WHERE WILL I HAVE THE TREATMENT?
You will be lying on a couch for the massage and sitting in a chair for lifestyle counselling.

WILL I BE CLOTHED?
You will need to strip to underwear for the massage, but you'll be covered with towels. Otherwise, you will remain fully clothed.

WHAT HAPPENS?
Expect careful questioning and pulse-taking (as with traditional Chinese medicine, Tibetan healing checks a variety of pulses to gauge health). In addition, the Tibetans use urine diagnosis for precise information on the person. The massage feels wonderful. It uses spiced or herbalized oils and works on the acupressure points to free blockages. You will be advised on diet and told which foods to avoid. Lifestyle tips may be given, too.

WILL IT HURT?
No, treatment is not painful. The massage is incredibly relaxing.

WILL ANYTHING STRANGE HAPPEN?
Not really. You may drift off to sleep during massage.

WILL I BE GIVEN ANYTHING TO TAKE?
If you see a fully qualified Tibetan physician, you will be given herbs, often in the form of tiny pills.

IS THERE ANY HOMEWORK?
Yes, you will be expected to make changes to your lifestyle and diet.

What's your Tibetan type?

Most people are a combination of types, but the following should give you a rough idea of which humor is dominating you at present.

AIR: Air causes stress. You may sweat very little and could suffer from insomnia, constipation, back pains, dry skin and stomach disorders. Your mind may flit from subject to subject. Symptoms include restlessness, dizziness, shivering, sighing, pain in the hips and shoulder blades, and humming in the ears.
DIAGNOSIS: A clear sign of unbalanced air is watery, almost transparent urine.
DIET TO BALANCE: Avoid cold foods such as salads and ice cream, or make sure you have a hot drink beforehand (such as ginger tea). Base your diet on chicken, meat broths, cheese, onions, carrots, garlic and spices, spinach and leafy greens.

BILE: Bile people often sweat quite a lot. They are precise, analytical people with good mental powers, but can be a little antisocial. They often wake up feeling bright and cheerful but by midday are feeling irritable. Their weak spot is their liver and they can easily overheat. When bile is out of balance, you could feel thirsty, have a bitter taste in your mouth, suffer pains in the upper body, feel feverish and have diarrhoea or vomiting.
DIAGNOSIS: Unbalanced bile is present if your urine is yellow or brownish in colour.
DIET TO BALANCE: Choose cool, light foods such as salads and yogurt, and drink plenty of cool water. Avoid hot, spicy foods, nuts, alcohol and red meat.

PHLEGM: Phlegmatic people are generally heavy; they have even, stable and (sometimes) stubborn personalities and avoid rows. They are prone to oversleeping and like an afternoon siesta. Their problems tend to be bronchial or in the kidneys. If phlegm is out of balance, you could feel lethargic and heavy. You may suffer frequent indigestion or belching, distention of the stomach and a feeling of coldness in the feet. You might put on weight or find it difficult to lose weight.
DIAGNOSIS: Disordered phlegm shows itself in very pale, foaming urine.
DIET TO BALANCE: Keep the digestion warm with spices such as ginger, cardamom and nutmeg. Fennel and peppermint will help the digestion, too. Avoid dairy, as it is mucus-producing, and don't eat too much fruit if you are trying to lose weight.

Tibetan tips for health problems

For anxiety and tension – rub either side of your breastbone.

For chesty/phlegmatic conditions – fill a bowl with hot water and add a few drops of ginger oil. Sit with your feet in it until the water is no longer hot, then massage your feet.

For combating stress and putting digestion back into balance – massage the soles of your feet in a circular motion.

For constipation – rub the base of the 'web' of skin at the point where your thumb and forefinger meet. Regularly drink hot water that has been boiled.

For general wellbeing – stand up straight with your arms outstretched, then start spinning slowly round in a clockwise direction (anticlockwise if you are in the southern hemisphere). Keep your eyes fixed on a spot straight ahead of you to minimize dizziness (as you turn round, fix your eyes back on that spot as quickly as possible). You will probably not be able to manage more than six turns to begin with. Practise every day and slowly build up speed, gradually working up to 12 repetitions (no more, or you will lose the energizing effect).

For hayfever – try taking a spoonful of honey every day for a month before the hayfever season starts.

For insomnia – put 2 or 3 drops of ginger essential oil in a base oil (almond is nice and light). Rub it into the soles of the feet before bedtime. Children will fall asleep if you massage the sides of their feet.

For mid-afternoon tiredness – try hot, sweet foods, such as honey in hot water.

4
Energy Medicine

As we have already seen, the ancients understood that we are not just flesh and bones; we are infused with a subtle form of energy that cannot be seen by the naked eye or under the microscope of science. For many years, complementary and alternative therapists have worked with this subtle energy and seen with their own eyes that, by working on the esoteric level, they could affect huge changes in the physical body. Scientists remained sceptical: no one had ever seen a meridian, an aura, a chakra, they argued. In recent years, however, more openminded investigation into this field has shown remarkable results: you can see the aura and the subtle energy pathways. It has been proven that healers can effect physical change.

We stand on the brink of an explosion in energy medicine. In the future, it will not seem strange to treat cancer with colour, rheumatism with sound. No one will scoff at the concept of flower essences shifting emotions, homoeopathy (where not a molecule of the original substance remains) curing eczema, or acupuncture reversing infertility.

The key to all these ideas lies in the concept of vital energy. Most people tend to think in terms of matter and energy as separate entities. Our bodies are matter: we feed them food which gives us the energy to power them – just as we feed a car fuel to make it move. But, according to the new field of quantum physics, the molecules that compose the physical human body are actually just a form of vibrating energy. In fact, Albert Einstein concluded that matter and energy were actually perfectly interchangeable.

Equally, everything around us is energy: it just vibrates at different frequencies. Just as X-rays, radio and television waves, ultrasonic waves and microwaves have different frequencies, so, too, do the various systems of the human body and the world around us. The cells of the body actually emit pulses of light which scientists surmise may be part of a sophisticated communication system to organize the actions of cells within each body system.

Once you take these ideas on board, the entire concept of energy medicine instantly makes sense. Directing a specific sound at a particular organ could bring it back in balance by a form of 'entrainment', encouraging the diseased part to vibrate at the right frequency again. A gem, flower or homeopathic remedy's vibrational signature could have the same effect.

Equally, once we recognize that we are powered by energy, it's a swift jump to recognize that energy isn't just physical: we talk about emotional energy; natural energy; spiritual energy; sexual energy. We must free ourselves from thinking on purely mechanical, tangible lines and see the world around us as energy vibrating at different frequencies, concepts such as feng shui, emotional healing, Tantra and contact beyond death all become quite possible.

The whole field is remarkably complex and astonishing. Fortunately, you do not need to be a quantum physicist to use energy medicine! It can help, however, to understand a few key concepts.

We humans possess several specialized systems that supply energy and information to the organs, tissues and cells of the body at a variety of levels. The various forms of energy medicine view these in different ways, but there are some basic concepts on which most agree.

Forms of vital energy

There are many forms of bioenergy in the human body: metabolic energy, bioelectrical energy and biophotonic energy, to name but a few that scientists are now researching to understand how cells communicate. For our purposes, however, we'll focus on that which is known as subtle, or vital, bioenergy (also known as subtle magnetic life energies). Why? Because these are the systems that we can most readily and easily influence for ourselves.

Qi (in the Chinese system) and prana (in the Indian) are the forms of energy with which you may be most familiar. Both the Chinese and Indians have been aware of the existence of subtle energy in the body and the environment for thousands of years – their whole systems of medicine are built upon it.

Although both forms of energy are described slightly differently, in reality, they are both ways of describing the energy that is absorbed from the environment around us, from the food we eat and the exercise we take. It can also be inherited from our parents. Qi flows through channels known as *meridians*, while prana flows through channels called the *nadis*, and also through the *chakras*.

Energy medicine also teaches that there are fields of energy that lie beyond our physical form. The best known is the 'aura' (which forms around the body), but there are also etheric energy (which keeps the physical body in correct shape), astral energy (which deals with emotional energy), mental energy (which governs intellect, creativity and thought) and higher spiritual energy or soul energy (which is said to hold our memories from lifetime to lifetime).

Let's take a closer look at some of these concepts.

Balance your Chakras for health and harmony

Eastern religions teach that the human body contains many spinning spheres of bioenergetic energy, known as *chakras*. The major ones run from the base of the spine to the crown of the head. While scientists insist chakras don't exist because they cannot be seen under the microscope, clairvoyants claim they can easily 'see' them. And the PIP scanner (see Electro-Crystal Therapy, page 235) which takes information from sound and light frequencies in the body now shows what the mystics have known of all along: oscillating spheres of energy in a vertical line down the body.

The chakras are precise monitors of our physical and mental wellbeing. Each chakra is said to spin at a different frequency and, when each one spins at its perfect frequency, the systems of the body radiate perfect health; emotions are centred and balanced and we enjoy optimum health and a deep sense of peace. It's a little like tuning into a radio station: if you're on the wrong frequency, the sound is distorted and unpleasant; once you hit the right frequency, it becomes clear as a bell. However, with all the stresses and strains of modern life, it is easy for the chakras to fall out of frequency. When this happens, we fall prey to illnesses, feel under par or lose our emotional equilibrium.

Each chakra governs different emotions and life issues. By visualizing and meditating on the chakras, you can learn a lot about yourself, increasing your self-knowledge. You can also use your chakras to 'tune in' to various issues or life lessons. For example, if you wanted to connect to the feeling of unconditional love, you would focus on your heart chakra, visualizing it as a beautiful, clear green wheel of energy, vibrating in your heart area.

The table opposite shows the main chakras, their colours and the areas they govern.

Healing the Chakras

In an ideal world, all our chakras would be balanced, each spinning equally. However, most of us have one or more centres out of equilibrium. Sometimes the body itself will give us clues: a sore throat can be an indication that the throat chakra needs attention, headaches may be a hint that we need to work on our brow chakra and constipation may nudge us into looking at our base.

CHAKRA	LOCATION	COLOUR	GOVERNS
Base	Base of spine	Red	The physical body, social position, survival
Genital	Genitals	Orange	Sensuality and sexuality, emotions
Solar plexus	Solar plexus	Yellow	Self-esteem, energy, confidence, will, inner power
Heart	Heart/chest	Green	Love, intimacy, balance, relationships
Throat	Throat	Blue	Communication and creativity
Brow	Forehead	Indigo	Imagination, intuition, dreams and insights
Crown	Top of the head	Violet	Understanding, connection and the divine

THE BASE CHAKRA: You need to reconnect with your body. Start by doing as much physical exercise as possible – choose a sport or activity you enjoy (maybe dance, aerobics, running or swimming). Try massage – find a professional aromatherapist or bodyworker, or ask a friend or partner to give you a massage. Yoga would be excellent, as it heals and balances all the chakras. Gardening and pottery are good grounding exercises if you have a deficiency of base chakra. On a psychological level, look at your early relationship with your mother: talk to her about it if you can. If it's painful, talk to a trained therapist or counsellor.

THE SACRAL CHAKRA: Learn to trust and enjoy your senses – feel the textures around you, listen to new music and sounds, look at nature and at art, and taste different foods and drinks. Dance can help to liberate this chakra, as can bodywork. Gently try to get in touch with your emotions (with professional help if necessary) to release any old feelings of hurt, anger and guilt.

THE SOLAR PLEXUS CHAKRA: Anyone with problems in this chakra would benefit from doing sit-ups (abdominal crunches) to strengthen that area. Martial arts such as judo or tai chi would be excellent. Psychotherapy can help you build up the necessary strength to release or contain any pent-up anger and strengthen your sense of autonomy.

THE HEART CHAKRA: Breathing exercises will help all those with problems in the heart chakra – join a yoga or chi kung class that teaches breathing. Start a journal, writing down all your feelings and thoughts honestly. Look at your relationships and try to free yourself from suppressed grief and loss (with professional help if necessary). Start to accept yourself – just as you are.

THE THROAT CHAKRA: If you are lacking in energy in your throat chakra, you need to use your voice: singing, chanting, humming, shouting – anything to release the voice. Sound therapy or voicework would be wonderful. If you have too much energy here, practise the art of silence and concentrate on what other people are saying. All problems in this chakra benefit from bodywork or massage to release tension in the neck and shoulders, or you could try the Alexander technique or Pilates. Write your thoughts and unspoken feelings in a journal; write letters (they don't have to be sent).

THE BROW CHAKRA: Try painting and drawing – use whatever materials and colours you like and paint whatever comes to mind. Look at your painting and see what emotions emerge. Write down and work with your dreams. Try meditation or autogenic training. Guided visualizations can be useful, as can hypnotherapy (but only with a qualified expert).

THE CROWN CHAKRA: Meditation could be very useful for you. Be open to new ideas and new information – don't dismiss things until you've tried them. Examine your attitudes to spirituality and religion. If you have an excess of crown chakra energy, you need to connect with your body and the earth – try physical exercise, massage or gardening. If you have a deficiency, open yourself up to the idea of spirituality, drop your cynicism and cultivate an open mind.

Psychoneurimmunology

Psychoneurimmunology concerns the mind's ability to effect change in the body. Only now is this being admitted (and often grudgingly) by Western doctors, but it has been widely practised for millennia by Eastern cultures. The Chinese alone have accumulated a vast reservoir of evidence linking the powers of body and mind, neurology and immunology, and have developed specific techniques for activating that link.

The principal technique in psychoneurimmunology is visualization. Patients are taught to focus their mind to visualize healing energy flowing into ailing organs, to dissolve tumours, repair tissue and so forth. Psychoneurimmunology will always work best if the image used has some meaning for you. One young boy with cancer imagined jet fighters zooming into his body to bomb the tumours. His strategy worked: the tumours shrank and disappeared without any recourse to chemotherapy, radiation or surgery.

Other people with cancer have taken a more literal (but still highly effective) tack. They visualized the cell membranes of the cancer cells within their bodies splitting (the problem with cancer cells is that their membranes stay intact so the immune system does not realize the body is under attack). This tactic has greatly improved the recovery and mortality rates of people with cancer. Others have helped themselves through chemotherapy by visualizing increased blood cell production while they are having the treatment.

Studies have shown that if people with broken bones visualize the bone mending and regrowing, it genuinely speeds the healing process.

Basically, we are what we think we are. While it is not fair to say that we totally create our own reality (although there is a school of thought that says that every illness we suffer is due to our negative thoughts!), we can certainly use the power of thought and visualization to effect changes in the body and to facilitate our own healing processes.

Do-it-yourself visualization

You can use visualization to help virtually any condition, for relieving stress or for emotional recovery. Try this:
1 Find somewhere quiet where you will not be disturbed. Make yourself comfortable, either on the floor (covered with a blanket if it is cool) or in a comfortable chair.
2 Close your eyes gently and breathe calmly and deeply. Allow as much air as possible to fill your lungs. Become aware of it flowing right down to the very bottom of your lungs.

3 Now take 12 conscious breaths. Each time you breathe in, imagine you are also inhaling total relaxation and calm. As you breathe out, all the stress and anxiety leaves your body.

4 Relax for a minute, feeling how much more relaxed and calm your body and mind feel.

5 Think of a wonderful place in which you feel safe, secure and very happy. It might be an actual place or an image of an ideal retreat, e.g. a cosy room with an armchair and fire, a beautiful desert island with the sun warming your body, or perhaps a dappled glade in a cool forest.

6 Explore all around your place: what does it look, smell and sound like? How does it feel (the warm sun on your skin, the rough texture of bark, the rub of a warm blanket)?

7 Know that this place is safe and sacred. It is a place of inner peace and inner healing. Anything can happen here. Feel all the stress and strain, all the negativity and morbid thoughts simply evaporating as you sit or lie here quietly. Feel your body become lighter, softer, warmer, more peaceful.

8 Now bring healing into your body and your life. Become aware of the area around your heart. Gradually it is being suffused with light, with healing energy. Feel the light spreading out through your whole body (you may feel warmth or coolness, or a kind of tingling). The light pinpoints any areas that need healing and you feel your body respond and change.

9 Stay in your special place, as long as you like. You may want to meditate quietly or just sit and enjoy the relaxation. Know that this place is always available for you.

10 Slowly bring yourself back to waking reality. Become aware of the room and your body. Move your fingers and toes. Give yourself a good stretch. Slowly open your eyes. Rest for a few minutes before you race back to normal life.

5
Homeopathy

How can a tiny, tasteless white pill that retains not even one molecule of the original substance from which it was derived have a profound effect on the body and mind? It's senseless if you take a mechanical view of the body. If we look at homeopathy as energy medicine, however, it no longer appears impossible.

Homeopathy is one of the fastest growing, and most trusted, systems of natural healthcare. In skilled hands, it can seem like a miracle. Results can often be very swift indeed, particularly for acute conditions. Chronic cases do take longer, but improvements can be sweeping.

Homeopathy was founded by Samuel Hahnemann in the late eighteenth century. He trained as a doctor, but was also a skilled chemist. Instinctively, he felt that the medicine he had been taught was not the answer; often it seemed to do more harm than good. Hahnemann felt that the approach was all wrong and that 'we should imitate nature, which sometimes cures a chronic disease by another and employ in the disease we wish to cure that medicine which is able to produce another very similar disease, and the former will be cured; *similia similibus'*.

The idea wasn't actually new. In the sixteenth century, Paracelsus taught that within each disease lies the key to its cure. Hahnemann and the ancient physicians also realized that to effect a long and lasting cure, you couldn't just cure the disease: you needed to cure the whole person. Then, of necessity, the disease would cure itself.

Hahnemann's breakthrough came with his observations on the effects of cinchona bark which, when it was given to healthy individuals, produced symptoms that were very similar to those of the dangerous malaria fever. However, when it was given to actual sufferers, it appeared to cure the fever. Out of this Hahnemann developed the main principles of homeopathy, testing numerous substances on himself to find out what symptoms they caused. He found, quite bafflingly, that the more dilute the form of the remedy, the more effective it became and, consequently, he began to dilute remedies more and more. He also discovered that there was no point in precisely matching a remedy to a particular disease or condition. Five patients with flu might need five different remedies simply because they would all have slightly different symptoms.

Homeopathy works, we believe, as a form of subtle energy healing. The water, in which the remedies are initially diluted, may extract and store a form of energy which can affect the human body and psyche. As the homeopathic remedy is being prepared and progressively diluted, the physical elements of the substance are removed, leaving their energetic qualities behind. Hahnemann believed the remedies worked very much like a classic immunization, by creating an artificial illness in the patient that stimulates the body's defences, which rise up to cure the original ailment. However, it seems that the remedy, rather than producing a physical reaction at a structural cell level, is producing a vibrational reaction, a vibrational illness to stimulate the body to heal at a vibrational level.

What can homeopathy help?

- Homeopathy can help virtually all conditions – in experienced hands, it can be used to treat everyone from newborn babies to the very elderly.
- Acute conditions such as bee stings, colds and injuries respond well and quickly.
- It has been proved very useful in chronic complaints including arthritis, rheumatism, PMS and menopausal problems, high and low blood pressure, digestive problems and infertility.
- Problems with a psychological aspect respond very well: depression, anxiety, insomnia and stress-related conditions. Some homeopaths have worked with psychiatrists treating patients with severe mental-health problems.
- Children and babies respond wonderfully. It can help to treat a huge range of problems, including ear infections, colic, eczema and asthma.
- Animals also respond well and many vets now use homeopathy as an adjunct to conventional medication.

What can I expect from a session?

WHERE WILL I HAVE THE TREATMENT?
You will be sitting in a chair in the homeopath's consulting room.

WILL I BE CLOTHED?
Yes, you will be fully clothed.

WHAT HAPPENS?
Basically you just talk! At your first (and longer) appointment, you will be asked for a full medical history, including dates of illnesses, accidents, operations etc. You will also be asked to describe your present problem in precise detail.

The homeopath will ask you a series of questions, some of which can seem quite odd. Expect to talk about your feelings, your childhood, your dreams, maybe even your thoughts about God. These allow the homeopath to build up a complete picture of you and help to find your ideal remedy.

Some homeopaths will give you a remedy at the end of the session; others will send the remedy to you later.

WILL IT HURT?
No, although painful emotions may emerge.

WILL ANYTHING STRANGE HAPPEN?
Sometimes homeopathy has curious effects. You may find you dream a lot more. You may also find that you feel worse in some way after taking the remedy – this is called an aggravation and shows the healing process is under way. It should not last long, but do always tell your homeopath if you are feeling uncomfortable.

WILL I BE GIVEN ANYTHING TO TAKE?
Yes, homeopathic remedies usually come in the form of tiny white pills or powders, which are virtually tasteless.

IS THERE ANY HOMEWORK?
No, although it is helpful if you make a note of how you feel between appointments, particularly any changes and any dreams.

Homeopathic first aid

Although, for best results, you should always see a professional homeopath, every home should have a basic homeopathic first-aid kit. These remedies can dramatically help everyday problems.

For most first-aid situations, obtain your remedies in the sixth potency (often labelled 6x). They are readily available from health food stores and chemist shops or pharmacies. Keep them away from perfumes and essential oils.

Arnica is the great shock remedy. Give it immediately after any kind of accident or shock, whether physical or emotional. It is also very useful after visits to the dentist, after operations and following childbirth because it is incredibly healing.

Arsenicum album is the first remedy to consider when there is any thought of food poisoning – when someone has eaten food that is off or tainted. The classic symptoms are restlessness and irritability, a feeling of desperation, feeling thirsty but wanting only small sips, and intense burning pains.

Belladonna is wonderful for fevers when the face is brightly flushed, for bursting headaches when the face is red, for sunstroke and for sore throats when the tonsils are enlarged and red. It is very useful for bringing down fevers in babies and children.

Calendula is generally used topically as a lotion or ointment. It is wonderful for any kind of wound or sore, or for soothing rough or chapped skin. Calendula promotes healing and lessens scarring.

Cantharis can help to soothe and heal cystitis. It is useful for any kind of burning pain, especially in the bladder or urethra when connected with urination.

Chamomilla is a classic remedy for teething babies – provided they are fractious and always asking for things, and then tossing them away. This remedy can also help if you've drunk too much coffee and is particularly useful for combating insomnia after an emotional upset.

Gelsemium is the great flu remedy – suitable for the typical variety of flu where you have shivers up and down the spine, an aching back and limbs, and a tight headache. You would not be thirsty.

Ignatia is the great grief counsellor. Give ignatia after any form of emotional shock, fright or grief. It is wonderful for helping with bereavement – not just for humans, but also for pets (remember that children often grieve terribly for lost pets).

Ledum is useful for old bruises and for puncture wounds such as insect stings, splinters or nails.

Nux vomica helps with the ill-effects of overeating or eating the wrong kinds of food; overindulging in alcohol or drugs; overstudying and overwork. Nux vomica is considered the great destresser.

Petroleum is useful for travel sickness of all kinds. Also useful for travel sickness is **tabacum**. Experiment to see which suits you best.

Rhus tox eases sprains of joints or tendons, and can be used after any form of overexertion or strain. It is very useful, with arnica, after surgical operations.

6 Healing

We can all heal. As Jesus said in the Bible, 'These things that I do, so can you do and more.' Unfortunately, few of us take it seriously. Yet many of us might be healing every day, without even knowing it. Some would say that every time a doctor or nurse touches a patient with care and concern they are performing a kind of healing. Parent do the same when they cuddle their child, or when they lay a soothing hand on the forehead or give a loving squeeze of the hand. Even total strangers can give the healing touch: some people simply shake your hand or put a hand on your shoulder and you can almost feel their energy leaping out at you. Healing can be simple: the mere touch of hands. Or it can be clothed in ceremony with recitations of prayers or the chanting of mantras. Which form you choose is up to you.

Healing certainly didn't begin in the Bible. Like so many other natural therapies, healing was a part of most ancient cultures. There is documentation which shows that the Chinese were practising it 5,000 years before the birth of Christ. The ancient Egyptians used it; so did the Greeks and Romans. In many cultures, the laying on of hands has been practised in a straight line from antiquity: both the Native American and the Australian Aboriginal cultures still practise healing in the ancient way.

In the West, however, healing has been rather frowned upon for some centuries, although it is now gaining popularity and credibility once again. In 1956, the British Medical Association (BMA) published a report entitled *Divine Healing and Co-operation between Doctors and Clergy*. The report stated quite clearly that 'through spiritual healing, recoveries take place that cannot be explained by medical science'. At the forefront of the new wave of healing is the National Federation of Spiritual Healers, whose members have been working for the past 30 years to establish bona-fide healing. They are non-denominational and bound by a strict code of ethics. Many hospitals now happily accept them into their wards when a patient asks for their services.

But what happens when someone heals? The process seems so simple. The healer either just touches the patient or hovers their hands above him or her. Some simply sit and think about the patient getting well – even though the patient is many miles away. How can it work? Many healers say that they are bringing their patients into a higher level of being, where they are in touch with the healing power of God or some higher force. Others think in more prosaic terms and say they are using a biomagnetic or bioelectrical energy and bringing the body into balance. However they describe it, what seems to be happening is that the energy system of the body is being balanced.

Many healers will insist that they do not actually heal, but that they merely open up the body so it can perform its own healing. The healer is merely there to act as a catalyst. This is one reason why it is important for the patient to have at least some form of faith in the process. Healers recognize the enormous untapped power of the mind and believe that, if the mind desires healing, the body will follow suit. Hence many healers will use creative visualization or encourage their patients to take responsibility for their own health, instigating changes in diet, exercise, mental attitude, stress relief and so on.

There is no doubt, however, that some people do seem to be 'tapped in' to some enormous fund of energy. They're a bit like live wires, literally buzzing with vital force. Kirlian photographs of healers' hands show bright, darting shoots of energy. And the PIP scanner used in electro-crystal therapy (see page 235) has filmed a healer working on a patient – as she put up her hands, clear shooting energy flew from her hands to the patient's body.

What can healing help?

- Many people turn to healing as a last-ditch attempt, when other therapies have failed.
- It is generally most successful when it prompts changes in the patient's lifestyle.
- People generally find they start to question their lifestyles and discover better ways to live.
- There have been cases of healing instigating almost miraculous cures – but it is unpredictable.
- Many people find healing a particularly soothing and relaxing form of stress relief.
- Because it is so gentle, this therapy is suitable for the very young, the very old and the very weak.
- Healing seems to help dying people – lessening pain and giving a sense of acceptance and peace.
- Animals also seem to respond well.

What can I expect from a session?

WHERE WILL I HAVE THE TREATMENT?
Usually you will be either sitting in a chair or lying on a couch in the healer's room.

WILL I BE CLOTHED?
Yes, you will be fully clothed.

WHAT HAPPENS?
Some healers will talk for a while before healing, using it as a chance to scan chakras (see page 41). You will then be asked to take off your shoes and jewellery, and then you will either lie on a couch or remain sitting in a comfortable chair.

Healers have different methods. Some will lay their hands gently on your body; others will have their hands hovering just over your body, working on the aura.

WILL IT HURT?
No, healing is totally painless. Usually you won't feel anything.

WILL ANYTHING STRANGE HAPPEN?
Some people feel energy moving in their body by tingling or shivering. Sometimes they can feel warmth or coolness coming from the healer's hands. Some people see colours or scenes from their lives.

WILL I BE GIVEN ANYTHING TO TAKE?
Not usually, although some healers do use flower remedies.

IS THERE ANY HOMEWORK?
It depends on your healer. Some healers will teach you visualization exercises or simple meditations.

Do-it-yourself healing

Anyone can learn healing touch – the process is incredibly simple, but will take time and practice to perfect. We will be looking at various types of healing and ways in which you can practise healing yourself and others throughout the book. But let's start now with some simple exercises to awaken your healing powers.

FEELING THE LINK BETWEEN MIND AND BODY
Before you start to heal, try the zero-balancing exercise on page 202, which should convince you that there is a definite link between your mind and your body.

FEELING YOUR OWN ENERGY
1 Rub your hands together quite vigorously for a few moments. Now hold them a few inches apart, as if you were holding a ball. You may feel a tingling or a warmth from your hands. 'Bounce' your hands and feel the energy change as your hands move closer and further away.
2 Now move your hands even further apart, as if you were holding, say, a football or volleyball.
3 Now imagine that in the centre of one palm is a circular patch that can transmit energy. Rub this area with the thumb of your other hand, imagining you are opening up this area. Then repeat on the other hand. If you have any religious or spiritual beliefs, you could ask for help in your healing quest.

SENDING HEALING ENERGY
1 Ask your subject to sit in a comfortable chair, then to relax, close his or her eyes and breathe naturally.
2 Stand with your feet shoulder-width apart. Let your shoulders relax and imagine there is a string gently tugging your head up to the ceiling. Breathe deeply and calmly, connecting with your heart chakra (imagine it pulsing with energy).
3 Now feel your crown chakra (at the top of your head) opening to let in healing energy. Visualize this energy flowing smoothly into your heart and then along your arms and into your fingers.
4 Now direct this energy where you feel it is needed. If you can sense that there is a particular place which needs attention, hold your hands either directly on that part or just above it.
5 If you are unsure where to heal, concentrate on the major chakra sites, starting with the base and moving up to the crown. Check the chart on page 41 for the various chakras. Visualize the healing energy streaming into each centre in turn. As you work, you might feel your hands become stiff or uncomfortable. Quietly shake them to release any negative energy you might have picked up while working. Every so often, pause and breathe to centre yourself.

7 Nutrition: Good Food

We are fed so much conflicting advice on diet that it's hard to sort the lean facts from the big fat fiction. It seems as though every day we read that we should be eating more protein or less protein; that we should give up all fat or that we should cut down on certain kinds. It can be so confusing that many people simply give up and eat what they like. Yet even a little (let alone too much) of what you fancy can be harmful to your health. Today, our food is so processed, so tampered with that you would be shocked to discover how little goodness it actually contains – and how much nastiness.

Almost all non-organic food is grown with pesticides of some kind. Many of these are health-threatening: some are carcinogenic (cause cancer); some are mutagenic (cause cells to mutate); others could be teratogenic (cause birth defects). The worldwide death rate from pesticide poisoning alone tops 200,000 a year, yet we still spray our crops.

Also causing concern is genetic modification (GM). Altering the genetic structure of a food to improve a particular quality is, warn some, an imprecise science with unpredictable outcomes. Bovine spongiform encephalopathy (BSE), or 'mad cow' disease, continues to pose a real concern, with fears that the disease which can be passed on to humans as variant Creutzfeldt-Jakob disease (vCJD) is on the increase.

Basic safety guidelines for a modern diet

- First and foremost, try to buy as much organic food as possible. It *is* more expensive, but prices are coming down.
- If you can't buy organic, always peel or skin non-organic vegetables and fruit to remove superficial additives (be aware that some pesticides will be absorbed into the food). Always buy organic meat – it's much better to have just a little organic meat than a large piece of non-organic.
- Pick food in season wherever possible. Food grown and harvested at its natural pace will have the most nutrients and vitality. Food grown out of season is usually forced with excess fertilizers and heavily treated with pesticides and fungicides. 'Baby' or miniature vegetables will have been heavily treated, too.
- Choose locally produced food which is less reliant on processing and additives to keep it looking fresh.
- Avoid foods with additives, colourings and preservatives wherever possible. This means all highly processed, convenience foods, including most canned, dried and packet foods, plus ready-made meals and 'fast foods'.
- Avoid smoked meats and fish, and steer clear of sausages and processed meats, which contain high levels of additives and potential carcinogens.
- Be wary of 'diet' foods, which often contain artificial sweeteners and other additives.
- Cut out (or cut right down on) sweets or candies. Most are packed full of artificial

colours, preservatives and other additives, which many people suspect of being prime factors in hyperactivity and allergic reactions in children.
- Cut down on red meat (except game), full-fat dairy produce and saturated fat. These can all contribute to heart failure.
- Try not to add salt to your food. Instead, use herbs and spices, or add celery, which has a naturally salty taste.

Glycaemic Index – the hidden factor

Research throughout the 1990s has shown that not all carbohydrates are created equal. For the most health benefits, we should be stoking up on foods with a low glycaemic index (i.e. foods that break down slowly, releasing glucose gradually into the body). Apparently, concentrating on these foods in our diet can improve heart conditions, give us more long-lasting energy and help us lose weight. On page 57, the wonder foods that you should include in your diet are listed.

WONDER FOODS
- whole cereal grains such as barley, whole wheat, cracked wheat (bulgur), oats and rolled oats (good for breakfast), and wholegrain breads
- dried pulses and legumes such as lentils, beans and dried peas. Use them as good sources of protein, in place of meat, in chillis, stews and casseroles
- fruit and vegetables – although be aware that potatoes have a high glycaemic index

Supplements – do we need them?

If you're eating a healthy diet, do you really need supplements? The shelves are brimming with vitamins, minerals, amino acids and herbal formulae, but are they truly necessary?

Sadly, many nutritionists now believe that we don't get the micronutrients we need from our daily diet. Few people enjoy the luxury of eating completely fresh, organic, additive-free food all the time. Plus, our modern, stressful lifestyle tends to strip vitamins and minerals from our bodies. Stress, pollution, smoking and alcohol can all scupper our best intentions. Hence, many experts now recommend taking a good-quality multivitamin and mineral compound as a safeguard against possible deficiencies. I think this is a good idea. Choose one from a reputable company (price will usually give a good indication – low-cost multis tend to be low quality): if in doubt, ask at your local health food store or consult your natural health practitioner.

If you are pregnant, you should not take a standard multi, but choose instead a specific antenatal one (ideally, consult a nutritional therapist). There are also now a broad range of multis for a range of people: children (a supplement can be very useful if you have a picky eater), teenagers, women (many find that it can help premenstrual syndrome (PMS) and other menstrual symptoms), sportspeople, menopausal women, and older people.

However, I would seriously warn against self-prescribing anything much more than a multicomplex. The biochemistry of micronutrients is indeed complex and you really need to consult a well-trained, experienced nutritional therapist if you feel that additional supplements would help.

The good-health diet

So, after you have cut all the baddies from your diet, what is left to eat? Fortunately, there is plenty of tasty food that should form the basis of your daily diet.

The World Health Organization (WHO) has come up with very simple guidelines based on universally agreed scientific principles. Interestingly, they reflect what most ancient medical philosophies have taught for centuries.

- Around half your daily intake of calories should come from complex carbohydrates (the solid, starchy foods such as bread, pasta, potatoes, cereals and rice). Ideally, choose the wholemeal or 'brown' versions of these, as they retain more nutrients, provide better fibre (which keeps your intestines healthy) and have a low glycaemic index (see page 54). Grains such as barley, millet, buckwheat and quinoa are also a good choice.
- Eat loads of fresh (ideally organic) fruit and vegetables – at least five portions a day (a portion is a piece of fruit, i.e. an apple or orange, or a serving of vegetables). Fruit and vegetables are packed with essential vitamins and minerals, including the disease-fighting antioxidants.
- Cut down on sugars – including syrups, fructose and sucrose (the so-called simple carbohydrates). Sugar simply isn't needed in a healthy diet. If you can't give up sugar (or sweet things) altogether, try to cut down or have a cake or chocolate as a special treat, rather than a daily snack.
- Cut down on saturated fat. Some fat is essential for health – and it's pretty hard to avoid fat entirely – but saturated fat puts us at risk from heart disease and some cancers. The main culprits are fried foods, some cuts of red meat (except game, which is surprisingly healthy) and full-fat dairy produce. Fish is great (oily fish such as herrings, mackerel and sardines do contain fat, but it's the healthy kind), so try to incorporate fish into your diet at least twice a week. Chicken and turkey are low-fat meats; seafood is also a good choice. Investigate vegetarian proteins such as tofu and Quorn, pulses, seeds and nuts.
- Experiment with herbs and spices. They have many health benefits, so get into the habit of adding some spice to your cooking. You will also find that you'll need less salt, sugar and fat because they give added interest to your food.

Nutritional therapy

The basic nutritional guidelines that have just been given are literally that – basic.

The cornerstone of all natural health thinking is that we are all individuals with individual needs. The food I thrive on might give you terrible indigestion; the diet that gives you masses of energy might make me put on weight. Equally, the diet that cures one person's arthritis might have no effect on someone else with the same condition. There are simply too many factors to take into consideration.

Nutritionists look at your entire lifestyle and make-up – not just what you eat, but how you work, how you sleep, what exercise you take, how you feel. The goal is to build a complete picture and then find a dietary and supplement programme to bring you back into health. It's also a process of education – finding out why you are imbalanced and how to correct it.

Nutritional therapy may seem like a new fad, but in fact the concept of curing illness with food is exceedingly ancient. Chinese and ayurvedic physicians would always look to diet first. Researchers in the twentieth century began to prove what the ancient sages knew through experience. Christian Eijkman, a Dutch doctor, found that prisoners in the East Indies who ate polished rice got the disease beriberi, while those who ate unrefined rice didn't. Polish biochemist Casimir Funk, working in London, discovered the element in rice husks that prevented the disease. He believed it belonged to a group of chemicals known as amines, so he coined the word 'vitamine', literally meaning an amine (essential) for life.

Nutritional therapy is not a quick fix and it can be tough going. To gain the best results, as with any therapy, you have to be committed and to make sacrifices for your health. You may well be told that you have to give up quite a number of foods for at least a month (to detect intolerances); you might equally be told some home truths about your lifestyle and urged to cut down on harmful practices.

The rewards, however, can be enormous. Many people find that their diet is at the root of some serious ailments.

What can nutritional therapy help?

- Arthritis and rheumatism respond well to nutritional therapy.
- Allergies and food intolerances can be factors in digestive problems, asthma, eczema and premenstrual syndrome (PMS) – nutritional therapy can help.
- Conditions with an emotional or psychological element such as depression, anxiety, insomnia, irritability and stress can often improve after an adjustment in diet or beginning correct supplementation, as can eating disorders.
- Children can respond well to dietary changes: hyperactivity can often be cured.
- Energy levels almost always increase, mood improves and people usually feel more relaxed.
- Almost all chronic conditions can be helped or alleviated in some way by nutritional therapy.

What can I expect from a session?

WHERE WILL I HAVE THE TREATMENT?
You will be sitting in a chair in the therapist's room.

WILL I BE CLOTHED?
Yes, you will be fully clothed.

WHAT HAPPENS?
First you will give answers to, or fill in, a detailed questionnaire, asking about all aspects of your health: history, current symptoms, energy levels, sleep, work and so on. Some nutritional therapists use kinesiology, dowsing or machines such as the Vega or BEST machine to detect allergies and intolerances, and check for deficiencies. Others will refer you for diagnostic tests.

From all this information, the therapist will work out what foods you should eat and what you should avoid, and also which supplements you need.

WILL IT HURT?
No, there's no pain involved – other than the pain of having to cut out foods you like and crave!

WILL ANYTHING STRANGE HAPPEN?
No, not at all. Nutritional therapy is a really practical, down-to-earth therapy.

WILL I BE GIVEN ANYTHING TO TAKE?
It is most probable that you will be prescribed supplements in the form of tablets or occasionally in liquid form.

IS THERE ANY HOMEWORK?
Yes, basically it's all down to you: having been told what to eat for good health, you are the one who has to stick to the guidelines.

8 Naturopathy

Naturopathy is to the West what ayurveda and traditional Chinese medicine are to the East – a gentle, nature-based, holistic health system that aims to put the whole body in balance. Many of the naturopathic 'cures' can be incorporated into everyday life with great ease. It's part of the reason why naturopaths see themselves as as much teachers as physicians.

The philosophy of naturopathy is very ancient. Hippocrates spoke of ponos, the body's incessant labour to restore itself to normal balance, while Aristotle spoke of the life force having a purpose beyond simply existing. Both insights chime with the naturopath's definition of naturopathy as 'a system of treatment which recognizes the vital curative force within the body'. In its current form, naturopathy has existed for more than 100 years. Its pioneers believed that ill health came about from a mix of hereditary factors, early environment (both before and after birth) and, most importantly, the lifestyle we lead. Most toxic of all is *mesotrophy*, the slow decline of the body's cells, in which poor diet is a factor.

The aim of naturopathy, then, is to allow the body to return to its natural equilibrium and its philosophy dictates that our bodies really do contain the wisdom and power to heal themselves – provided we help them and don't interfere too much. Readjusting our entire lifestyles can be unpleasant, if not downright painful, and naturopathy is certainly no easy option. Naturopaths use osteopathy to correct structural problems. Diet forms a large part of treatment, righting the biochemical balance of the body. Naturopaths also recognize the importance of mental and emotional health. Equally important is the patient's energy or vitality. The most natural cures available are favoured: fresh air and sunlight; fasting and a fresh, pure diet; relaxation and psychological counselling; and, very importantly, the healing power of water.

Some naturopaths are purists and work only with these basic tools. Others have incorporated other disciplines. Most naturopaths are masters of many arts, using herbalism, homeopathy and acupuncture in addition.

What can naturopathy help?

- Virtually all chronic diseases respond well to naturopathy.
- It has particular success with rheumatic and arthritic conditions.
- Hypertension and allergic and fatigue conditions often improve.
- It can be very helpful in promoting weight loss.
- Skin conditions can disappear or diminish.

What can I expect from a session?

WHERE WILL I HAVE THE TREATMENT?
It depends. You will sit in a chair for the initial consultation. You may lie on a couch for osteopathy or some forms of hydrotherapy; other forms are carried out in a bath, shower or pool.

WILL I BE CLOTHED?
You will be fully clothed for the initial consultation. You would strip to underwear for osteopathy and be naked for some hydrotherapy.

WHAT HAPPENS?
The initial consultation will seem quite medical in its approach and, if you have a serious medical condition, expect to be sent for X-rays, ECGs or blood tests. You may be tested for allergies with a Vega machine. Diet and exercise regimes will then be prescribed. If hydrotherapy is required, you may find yourself being hosed alternately with hot and cold water; lying in therapeutic mud; sitting in a steam 'pod'; or having hot-wax treatments on hands, feet or knees. Constitutional hydrotherapy involves lying on a couch while hot and cold towels are placed alternately over your body.

WILL IT HURT?
Some of the treatments are quite stringent and uncomfortable – although not painful.

WILL ANYTHING STRANGE HAPPEN?
Many hydrotherapy treatments can seem peculiar to begin with.

WILL I BE GIVEN ANYTHING TO TAKE?
Diet will always be a factor. If your naturopath also uses other disciplines, you might be given herbs or homeopathic remedies.

IS THERE ANY HOMEWORK?
Yes, lots. Naturopathy requires a lot of hard work – shifting diet, doing exercise, relinquishing bad habits.

Do-it-yourself naturopathy

Water therapy is intrinsic to naturopathy. It's cheap, it's easy to administer and it's literally on tap. There's no excuse for not borrowing a few tips from naturopaths and extending your use of water beyond the usual glass of water to drink and daily bath or shower to get clean. Naturopaths use water in the treatment of injuries, to relieve pain, to reduce fever, as a stimulant *and* a relaxant, and even as an anaesthetic. The following ideas should get you started on your own hydrotherapy.

SALT MASSAGE BATH
If you are feeling low or lacking in energy, this is an essential. It helps the circulation, is useful in easing rheumatic pain and will also get rid of all your dead skin, leaving your body feeling smooth and silky. It's also very simple to do.
   It is possible to stop a cold in its tracks this way, but don't do so if your skin is broken – it will sting unbearably.
CAUTION: do not try this if you have high blood pressure or a heart condition.
• Make a slushy paste with salt and warm water. If you can use sea salt, so much the better.
• Apply it all over your body, using circular movements.
• Now get into a bath filled with quite warm to hot water and soak for about 20 minutes.

APPLE CIDER VINEGAR BATH
This is a wonderful tonic if you're feeling tired and is also a prime detoxifier. It is soothing in summer if you are suffering from sunburn or have itchy skin.
CAUTION: do not try this if you have high blood pressure or a heart condition.
• Pour a little apple cider vinegar onto your hands and splash it all over your body.
• Now add a cupful of the vinegar to a warm-to-hot (but not scalding) bath and soak for a while.

MOOR BATH
A mud preparation from Austria containing literally hundreds of minerals and phytonutrients, this is a popular choice among naturopaths and usually readily available from health stores. It promotes deep relaxation and sound sleep. It has also been used medicinally for rheumatic conditions with very good results.
- Pour the suggested amount (see bottle) into a warm but not hot bath. Allow yourself to soak for about 20 minutes.
- Pat yourself gently dry and wrap yourself in a towel. Lie down and relax for at least an hour.

BODY PACK
You will need to enlist the help of a friend for this powerful treatment. Body packs work like a kind of sauna or steam – eliminating toxic waste through sweating.
- Immerse a cotton sheet totally in cold water, then wring it out, leaving it damp. The sheet shouldn't drip, yet needs to be cold to the touch.
- Spread the sheet over a bed or couch (you may wish to put down a plastic sheet underneath) and lie down on it.
- Place three hot-water bottles inside the sheet – one by your feet, one at your waist and one near your chest.
- Have someone wrap the ends of the sheet firmly around you and the hot-water bottles so you are covered from your neck down to your feet. You are now encased in your individual private steam 'room'.
- Relax like this for at least 3 hours. You will start to sweat profusely within 10 to 15 minutes, but the treatment is very relaxing and you will most likely fall asleep. By the end, the sheet will be almost dry and may be discoloured from the eliminated toxins. You will need to wash it before reusing it.

EPSOM SALTS BATH
Have this bath just before going to bed. Epsom salts induce prodigious perspiration and so are superlative for sweating out toxins. This bath is also very useful for rheumatic conditions and can help fend off infections, colds and flu as well.
CAUTION: avoid if you have heart trouble, if you are diabetic or if you are feeling tired or weak.
- Dissolve about 450 g (1 lb) of Epsom salts in a warm bath. (You can work up to this amount slowly over a week or two.)
- Relax for about 20 minutes. Drink a hot herbal tea (thyme or peppermint would be ideal) to increase perspiration and replace any lost fluids.
- Take care as you get out of the bath – you may feel light-headed.
- Do not rub yourself dry. Wrap up in several large towels and go to bed. Wrap your feet up warmly.
- In the morning, or when you wake, sponge yourself down with warm water. Rub your body vigorously dry.

Juicing

Naturopaths swear by freshly made fruit and vegetable juices. But just why are juices so wonderful? Fruits and vegetables are rich in micronutrients which have profound healing properties. Many of them actively encourage elimination. The majority of vegetables are highly alkaline in their nature and possess the ability to bind acids and eliminate them through the kidneys and urine. So juicing is ideal for anyone suffering from 'acid' conditions such as rheumatism and arthritis – provided, of course, you avoid citrus fruits, which exacerbate these conditions.
  Some naturopaths say that a day a week on a diet of vegetable juices will be bene-

ficial to almost anyone (see under fasting on page 67 for exceptions and always check with your doctor first). If you do decide on a juice-only day, you should have from 500–700 ml (½–¾ pint) up to a litre (2 pints) of fresh juice. For maximum, make several batches of juice over the day. Sip the juice slowly throughout the day – don't slurp it all down. Also, drink plenty of fresh water – either at room temperature or warm.

Juices for specific conditions

Certain combinations of juices are renowned for their healing and healthful properties.

ARTHRITIS carrot, celery and cabbage juice.

ASTHMA AND CATARRHAL CONDITIONS carrot and radish juice.

CONSTIPATION cabbage, spinach, celery and lemon juice.

HIGH BLOOD PRESSURE celery, beetroot and carrot juice.

LOW BLOOD PRESSURE carrot, beetroot and dandelion juice.

SKIN CONDITIONS carrot, beetroot and celery juice.

SORE THROATS, COLDS AND FLU lemon, lime and pineapple juice.

TO HELP YOU SLEEP celery juice.

TO OPEN UP SINUSES AND AIR PASSAGES horseradish and lemon juice (125 g/4 oz)· of horseradish and 60 g/2o z of lemon juice, combined with a teaspoon of garlic juice and a tablespoon of honey – take a teaspoonful four times daily).

TO SOOTHE THE NERVES lemon and lime juice.

The juices

Choose fresh, organic vegetables and fruit – ideally those in season. You will need a juicer for these recipes; follow the manufacturer's instructions for use.

Carrot juice is pleasant to drink and one of the best juices to start with if you're new to juicing. It really packs a good healthy punch, too.
- Carrot juice affects the mucus membranes of the body and stimulates blood circulation in the stomach and intestines.
- It is good for constipation, diarrhoea and digestive problems.
- When poor digestion is sorted out, other problems often disappear – headaches, eczema and bad skin can all vanish when the digestion is functioning properly.
- Carrot juice is refreshing and soothing, and helps the body battle against infectious diseases.
- Packed full of antioxidant vitamins, it fights the free radicals that cause disease and ageing.
- Its rich supplies of carotene (provitamin A) are necessary for eyesight and stimulate the production of rhodopsin (visual purple), lack of which causes night blindness.
- Carrot juice is also supposed to help regulate your weight and to give you a beautiful complexion.

Beetroot juice, with its dark purple colour, may look rather unappetizing, but don't let its appearance put you off as it is very beneficial to the health.

- Beetroot contains betaine, which stimulates the function of the liver cells, protecting the liver and bile ducts, and encouraging detoxification.
- Just 100 ml (4 fl oz) of beetroot juice contains 5 mg of iron, as well as trace elements that encourage iron's absorption in the blood.
- Everyone can benefit from beetroot juice, but it is particularly recommended in the first 2 years of life, during puberty, during pregnancy, when breastfeeding and during menopause. Children from 6 months to 2 years need only a teaspoon of juice before meals.

NOTE: beetroot juice is high in sugars. Seek expert advice about its use if you suffer from diabetes or blood glucose problems.

Celery juice tastes a bit salty when drunk on its own, but you can easily mix it with other vegetables to add flavour and give additional health benefits.
- Celery is alkaline and encourages elimination, and hence is recommended for any diseases or problems connected with an accumulation of wastes and toxins, such as arthritic and rheumatic ailments.
- Celery juice also regulates the water balance in the body and is superb for elderly people.

Apple juice is a wonderful source of vitamins, minerals and trace elements. A few apples juiced a day certainly do help keep the doctor away.
- Apples are astringent and can help alleviate diarrhoea.
- They promote elimination of excess fluid and toxins, so are good for arthritis, skin problems and fluid retention.
- Take apple juice when you're feeling under par – it speeds recovery from colds and coughs, and eases catarrh and sinusitis.
- Apples are cooling and so useful in cases of inflammation.
- They can help regulate blood sugar and cholesterol levels, and blood pressure.

Watercress juice is peppery and tangy, and a potent tonic. The plant draws a multitude of vital elements from the soil. You can combine it with other juices if you find the taste too strong.
- Watercress is a superb antiseptic and detoxifier. It is rich in vitamins A, C and E, and the minerals iron, potassium, zinc and calcium.
- Take watercress when you have chest infections, coughs and bronchitis – it is a good expectorant.
- Watercress juice cleanses the blood and so can be helpful in treating arthritis, gout and rheumatism.
- Watercress may help premenstrual syndrome (PMS).
- It is a tonic for the digestion, circulation, kidneys and bladder.

Apricot juice is sweet and delicious, and combines well with less palatable ingredients.
- Apricots are natural laxatives and are therefore wonderful for constipation. Children usually love the taste, so it can be very useful when encouraging them to drink juice.
- Apricots are high in betacarotene, which is protective against lung, skin and pancreatic cancers. If you smoke, you should certainly up your intake of apricots.
- They are very nourishing and easily digested, so are ideal for anyone feeling tired and weak; they are a great convalescence food and ideal for pregnant women, the elderly and children.

CAUTION: some people are allergic to apricots. If you are buying dried apricots, always choose the unsulphured variety as the sulphur used in preserving can also cause allergies.

Detoxifying

Do we need to detoxify? Sadly, we do. Our world is so polluted that our bodies can benefit greatly from even a short period of rest and recuperation. It need not be Draconian. A few simple changes can have profound effects. Try the following.

1 Alcohol is a big toxic enemy. Cut down your intake as much as possible. Try drinking wine diluted with water if you need to drink socially.

2 If you smoke, do try to give up – you will be doing your body a huge favour. Acupuncture and hypnotherapy can help.

3 Cut down on tea and coffee. To avoid headaches and other side effects of caffeine withdrawal, take it slowly, reducing your intake by a cup a day. Try caffeine-free herbal teas and drinks instead, or hot ginseng essence with honey for a real energy boost.

4 Drink water – lots of it – throughout the day. It cleanses the system, helps flush out toxins and has the added bonus of making you feel less hungry if you're trying to lose weight.

5 Clean up your diet. Highly processed foods and 'junk' foods are full of toxic additives. Follow the guidelines on page 57 and eat as pure and as organic a diet as you can.

6 Treat yourself to a good-quality juicer and enjoy nourishing, energy-packed fresh fruit and vegetable juices for mid-morning and mid-afternoon treats. It's worth buying a top-of-the-range model with easy cleaning facilities.

7 Start a regime of skin brushing before your shower or bath to stimulate the flow of lymph and promote good circulation. Use either a damp flannel with a bicarbonate-and-salt mixture or a special skin brush. Start by moving from the feet up the legs towards the back of the knees, then up the thighs to the groin. From the fingers, brush arms towards the armpits, then gently from the neck towards the heart. Then do the back and torso, again always towards the heart. Avoid areas that are broken, tender or irritated. Start with gentle movements, building up to gentle but firm pressure.

8 Give yourself a detox-diet weekend.
   • Breakfast one type of fruit (as much as you like), hot water or herbal tea.
   • Mid-morning snack fresh fruit or vegetable juice.
   • Lunch salad of raw vegetables, bean sprouts and almonds (season with orange or lemon juice, garlic and ginger).
   • Afternoon snack fruit.
   • Evening meal vegetable soup, salad, steamed vegetables. Drink plenty of water throughout the day.

9 Exercise. All aerobic exercise (jogging, cycling, swimming, stair climbing, brisk walking and so on) helps to maintain the lymphatic flow. Don't conserve energy – run up the stairs, use housework as exercise (scrub to the beat), go to the gym or take a brisk walk at lunchtime, rather than hailing the sandwich trolley from your desk. Probably the best exercise of all for your lymphatic system is rebounding (bouncing on a small trampoline), which need not be expensive. Just 20 minutes a day will really help your detoxifying (and also give you a good aerobic workout).

10 Treat yourself to a massage. Manual lymphatic drainage (see pages 226–7) by a professional is the ideal, but any massage using effluage (firm stroking movements, always in the direction of the heart) is good for detoxifying (and is destressing as well). If you can't afford regular professional massages, form a duo with your partner or a friend and learn how to massage (MLD practitioners will teach you the basic technique or you can learn ordinary massage from videos or on short workshops). Then you can trade massages.

11 Breathe deeply and calmly. Try to set aside 10 minutes each day to concentrate on breathing slowly, rhythmically and deeply, sending air into every cell of your body in order to oxygenate the blood.

- Sit comfortably and start by breathing in while slowly counting in your head to four. Hold for a count of four, then release to the count of four.
- When that feels comfortable, count up to six, hold for six and release for six. Eventually, you should feel able to breathe in to eight, hold for eight and release for eight.

For more breathing exercises, see pages 80–1.

Fasting

All over the world, religions have espoused the spiritual benefits of purifying and castigating the body by withholding food. In medieval times, fasting was a way of life. Today, few people see of fasting as primarily a religious experience and it certainly isn't regarded as punishment: fasters are usually seeking a healthier body, brighter mind and clearer emotions.

The traditional fast is pretty tough: you just drink water and that is all. Although this is still practised in naturopathy, many people now practise modified fasts, drinking just juice or eating one type of fruit, usually apples or grapes.

There is evidence supporting the value of periodic, sensible fasting. Research has been carried out since 1880 and, since then, medical journals have carried occasional reports on the use of fasting for the treatment of obesity, eczema, irritable bowel syndrome, bronchial asthma, depression and even schizophrenia. Today, however, most people use it as preventative medicine.

The digestive system uses up to 30 per cent of the total energy produced by the body; by putting the system into a state of rest, we help the body to concentrate on detoxification and healing. On a health level, naturopaths say that fasting can improve your immune function and allow your body a decent chance to deal with its problems; on a beauty level, fasting can make your skin look fresher and more toned, your eyes brighter and your hair more lush.

Fasting is not, however, a good way to lose weight. Six hours after the last meal, the body starts to use glycogen (the carbohydrate stored in the liver and muscles) as its energy source. After 24 hours, your body takes its energy not just from stored fat, but also from the breakdown of muscle. After several days, your metabolism will slow to conserve energy and, if you fast for too long, the ability to digest food may be impaired or lost entirely because the stomach gradually stops secreting digestive juices. Sex hormones are no longer produced and your body loses its ability to fight infection.

CAUTION: Fasting is not for everyone. If in doubt, don't do it. It is distinctly not advised if you are pregnant or breastfeeding, if you have any medical condition and particularly if you have any eating disorder. Always ask your doctor or a qualified practitioner and don't fast unsupervised for more than 24 hours.

9 Herbalism

We merrily add herbs to our cooking without a second thought. We certainly don't stop to think about their healing virtues! Yet herbs have been used for centuries as a potent form of medicine. Discovering the healing power of herbs can be a fascinating journey – and can have deep, long-lasting effects.

It is safe to say that herbalism is probably the very oldest of all forms of medicine. It doesn't take much imagination to think that the early hunter–gatherer societies would have discovered, through trial and error, that not only were certain plants good to eat, but that some also had curative powers.

Take any ancient culture and you are bound to find it has a tradition of herbalism. In fact, the herbal tradition stayed firmly centre stage until the advent of modern chemical medicines. Now research is discovering that herbs can be as effective as synthetic preparations – and often more so.

Herbal medicines work on a simple biochemical level. They trigger neurochemical reactions in the body and so directly affect its organs and systems. Basically, they fulfil three classic functions: they cleanse, they heal and they nourish.

First, before a body can bring itself to health, it needs to rid itself of the toxins and dead and decaying matter that litter the body. Herbs can be used as diuretics, laxatives and blood purifiers to help the processes of elimination and detoxification. The next step is to escort the body back to optimum health: herbs are used to stimulate the body's own self-healing powers and to attack the underlying causes of illness. Thirdly, herbs are used to tone the various organs and to nourish all the systems of the body, helping it keep on an even, healthy keel.

The aim is that, by taking the herbs over a period of time in moderate doses, the biochemical responses of the body will become automatic and it will start fending for itself again, even when you stop taking the herbs.

Famous herbal healers

Several herbs have become specially famous in recent years. The following are some you may have heard of:

Aloe vera is a wonderful home first-aid remedy for burns, wounds and sunburn. Buy the gel for topical application. It is also marvellous for insect bites and fungal infections.

Echinacea (purple coneflower) is now well known as a cure-all for colds, flu and other infections. Buy in capsule form and take three 200 mg tablets up to three times a day as soon as you feel yourself coming down with an infection. Do not take echinacea on a longstanding, ongoing basis – use it only as a short course.

Ginkgo is excellent for improving circulation. It is a useful herb for people with diabetes, eye problems, heart conditions and memory loss. However, you should always see a medical herbalist for prescription.

Milk thistle is a great cleansing herb and very useful if you have been living the high life and need to give your liver some TLC! It is helpful in detoxifying for the same reason.

St John's wort (hypericum) is one of the most popular herbs. It is mainly taken for depression and has proven as effective as conventional antidepressants for many people. However, St John's wort should always be taken under the guidance of a professional herbalist, as it can have side effects and may interfere with the efficacy of other drugs.

Wild yam is a herb that has hit the headlines because of its beneficial effects on menopausal women. Wild yam is believed to be progesteronic (supportive of the body's progesterone cycle), but does not, as commonly supposed, actually contain progesterone in it. See a herbalist if you think that this would be helpful for you.

Saw palmetto is a superb herb for prostate conditions. It's an excellent male tonic herb and careful supplementation can prevent or halt the progression of benign prostatic hyperplasia (BPH). See a herbalist for prescription.

What can herbalism help?

- Herbalism is used for a variety of acute and chronic conditions.
- Herbs can support detoxifying – cleansing and purifying the body.
- Herbal tonics can give a boost and improve energy levels.
- Herbs can be used to ease aches and pains; headaches and migraines; and all manner of eye, ear, nose and throat problems. Skin problems respond well, too.
- Allergic conditions can often be alleviated.
- Urinary disorders, gynaecological problems and digestive problems respond appreciably.
- Herbs can help respiratory and circulation problems.
- Herbs can boost the immune system and so help resist infections.
- Herbs can be very useful in pregnancy and childbirth, and can also be used to treat children.

What can I expect from a session?

WHERE WILL I HAVE THE TREATMENT?
You will be sitting in a chair in the herbalist's room.

WILL I BE CLOTHED?
You will usually remain fully clothed, although some clothes may need to be removed for examination purposes.

WHAT HAPPENS?
Expect a physical check-up and also to answer questions about your symptoms and medical history (emotional life, work, sleep, family history, and so on). It's a very detailed consultation. Your blood pressure may be taken, and heart and chest listened to with a stethoscope. You may have your ears, nose, throat and eyes examined; your abdomen may be palpated (gently prodded and felt) to gauge bowel tone. If necessary, blood tests are given.

WILL IT HURT?
No, although herbal tinctures are very bitter and often unpleasant.

WILL ANYTHING STRANGE HAPPEN?
No, herbalism is a very straightforward therapy – the most akin of all therapies to a visit to an orthodox medical doctor.

WILL I BE GIVEN ANYTHING TO TAKE?

Yes, herbs will be prescribed – usually in tincture form (you dilute them in water and swallow). You may be given dried herbs with which to make an infusion (steeped in boiling water like tea) or a decoction (boiled down into a concentrate). Sometimes pills, lotions and creams are prescribed.

IS THERE ANY HOMEWORK?

You will often be given guidelines for healthier living and diet, and exercise may be suggested.

Healing herbs – safe do-it-yourself remedies

Generally speaking, you should always consult a well-qualified herbalist. Herbs are powerful medicines and should not be treated lightly. Some can interfere with other medications; others should not be taken during pregnancy or if you have high or low blood pressure.

However, the following herbs can be used safely by most people (where there are contraindications, these are stated). Most can be grown in your garden.

To use, place 30 g (1 oz) of the dried herb or 75 g (2½ oz) of the fresh herb in a teapot or jug (pitcher). Pour over 500 ml (1 pint) of boiled water (it should have been freshly boiled, but left to stand for a few moments so that it is no longer bubbling). Leave for 10 minutes and then strain. Take the herb in three equal doses throughout the day.

Camomile is your best friend if you're stressed or suffer from insomnia. Drink a cup of camomile tea at night to ease you to sleep. Camomile will also soothe indigestion, stimulate a poor appetite and soothe an irritable bowel. (**NOTE:** avoid during pregnancy.)

Fennel is the perfect after-dinner digestive. Drink fennel for all kinds of digestive problems, from flatulence to indigestion. (**NOTE:** avoid during pregnancy.)

Ginger is a safe remedy for morning sickness and is also wonderful for indigestion, nausea and travel sickness.

Hops are another great insomnia aid and are often combined with valerian, vervain, camomile or meadowsweet in herbal teas designed to help you get a good night's sleep. (**NOTE:** avoid if you suffer from depression.)

Lemon balm can help revive you if you're feeling worn out and depressed. It will also help if you feel you are starting to come down with a cold or flu.

Mint (shown opposite) is another great stomach soother that is wonderful for nausea, travel sickness, indigestion and flatulence. It can ease headaches and is a good pick-me-up. (**NOTE:** mint can reduce milk flow, so avoid if breastfeeding.)

Nettle is the great cleanser; it stimulates the circulation and makes a superb tonic. It can be very helpful in cleansing the system if you are suffering from conditions such as arthritis, rheumatism and eczema.

10 Exercise

Exercise is an essential part of the good health equation. Regular exercise keeps your heart and lungs working at optimum levels and helps ward off heart disease. Stress levels drop when you exercise, so you will come away from a workout or sports game feeling a general lift in mood. Regular exercise can perk up your sex life and give you a good night's sleep; it can also help control blood pressure and boost your immune system.

Of course, if you are concerned about your weight, beginning to exercise is the very best move you can make. Excess flab disappears when you start to work out; your body becomes more flexible and more toned. The more muscle you have, the more fat you burn: you simply can't help but get slimmer and trimmer.

Motivate yourself

There's really no excuse for not exercising – yet we manage to invent plenty! It can be tough to get started, so many of us simply don't bother. If you commit to a regular exercise programme, however, you will begin to notice changes quite swiftly. At first, you might be out of breath after just two minutes of jogging or cycling. But rest assured, after a few sessions, you will be up to a good 6 minutes and, within 6 weeks, should be able to breeze through 30!

The following exercise tips will help you boost your motivation levels.

What do you want from exercise?

Check that you're matching your exercise with your goals.
- If you want to change your shape and improve your appearance, go for activities that deliver noticeable results: weight training; circuit training, yoga and Pilates will all change your body shape.
- If you want to lose weight, you need moderately high-intensity sports such as running, stepping, aerobics, fast cycling, brisk walking and power yoga.
- If you want to get healthy without strain, go for low-impact aerobics, swimming, cycling and walking.
- If you want to beat stress, try yoga, tai chi, boxing or skating, plus sports that allow you to go on automatic pilot such as running, walking and swimming.

Find an expert

If you can, enlist the help of an expert to get you on the right track. A good gym, for instance, should give you a fitness assessment, a tailor-made programme and bags of encouragement along the way. If you're on your own, you'll probably succeed through trial and error. If you don't like one kind of exercise or routine, or you don't get results after giving it your best shot (it will take 6 weeks of regular sessions to notice a significant difference), change. If that doesn't work, change again. Obviously, you need to give any programme a fighting chance, but don't ever force yourself to do something you hate. If exercise is going to work for you, it has to be enjoyable or, at the very least, challenging!

Start small

If you haven't exercised before or not for a long time (and especially if you're returning to exercise after pregnancy), take it easy. If you can get yourself past the first week, you've passed the period in which half of all drop-outs occur. If you work out regularly for six months, you're likely to have created a long-lasting habit. Grin and bear it for that first week (yes, it will be tough) and then it will start to get easier.

The really brilliant thing about exercising regularly is that you soon notice the results. There is nothing more motivating than looking in the mirror and seeing yourself definitely firmer; there is nothing better than seeing a thigh stop wobbling and start rippling.

Discover your fitness personality

You love sushi, your best friend hates it. So, where is it written in stone that we should all be doing step and loving it? Just because all your friends adore swimming, why should you? There are a million and one ways of exercising, so you simply need to find those that a) you enjoy and b) fit in with your lifestyle – then the odds are that you'll keep them up. The following are just a few ideas of how you can tailor your exercise regime to suit your personality and lifestyle.

- **You're a workaholic** You can't afford the luxury of exercising. But remember that exercise relieves stress and will help you become more energized, more focused, more creative. Try running or cycling to and from work. Visit the gym or fit in a yoga class at lunch-time – it will make you more productive in the afternoon. If you're a competitive type, play squash or badminton with colleagues.
- **You're a stressed-out mum** You don't have time to think, let alone exercise. Remember first of all that exercise will relieve the stress and make you (and, by extension, your child) calmer. And, if you feel dead on your feet, it will actually give you more energy. Researchers have compared the effects of a sugary snack with a 10-minute brisk walk on volunteers' moods. The snack certainly gave an instant boost of feelgood factor, but the effects swiftly wore off, leaving the volunteers feeling even worse than before. The exercisers, meanwhile, were still feeling great up to two hours afterwards. Many gyms and local fitness centres now have childminding facilities, so check them out, or get together with some friends, hire a trainer and organize your own aerobics class or circuit training. Don't have time? Involve the whole family in exercise: play with your kids (that can be serious exercise in its own right) or bundle everyone off to the park, the boating pond, the ice rink, the swimming pool … It doesn't have to be the gym or a formal class – just get moving.
- **You see exercise as one long, dreary chore** You need variety and to pick out activities that don't really seem like exercise. Forget the gym and formal classes – think laterally: rollerblading, dancing, trampolining, horse riding, surfing. What did you enjoy doing when you were a child? See if it still gives you a buzz.
- **You get bored exercising on your own** Who says you have to pound the lonely Stairmaster? One of the best ways to motivate yourself is to train with a friend. It's much more fun and, if you like jogging or running, it's much safer, too. If your resolve starts to slip and you're tempted to opt out, you'll not only let yourself down, you'll also letting your friend down (guilt can be a powerful motivator). Apparently, at least 90 per cent of exercisers prefer to work out with other people, rather than solo – so you're not alone. No friends willing to play the game? Join a circuit class or put your name down for a league.

- **You like a bit of excitement** We often forget that team sports count as exercise, too. Remember netball? Hockey, volleyball, softball, football, basketball? Why not? You'll meet new people, have fun and get fit almost by accident.
- **You feel self-conscious about your body and your abilities** Choose something strictly non-competitive. Yoga is ideal because you focus solely on what you are doing. Sometimes you even have to keep your eyes shut! Forget a skimpy leotard – most people wear leggings or sweatpants and a baggy T-shirt. And yoga is a wonderful toner – it gives you beautiful, long, lean muscles.

Stretching

Everyone should make time to stretch. Stretching is simplicity itself, yet it is absolutely wonderful for both body and mind. If you carry out a careful stretch routine before and after exercise or sports, you will help to protect your muscles and joints from injury. If you spend your days stuck at a desk or behind the wheel of a car, stretching can release stress and help relax any tense muscles.

Stretching will also improve your posture and you will be far less likely to suffer from neck, shoulder and back pain, headaches and bad digestion.

Virtually anyone can follow a simple stretch routine. However, if you do suffer from a bad back, you should seek professional advice before stretching.

Try to make the simple stretch routine opposite a daily habit. Practise it in the morning to give your body a wake-up call and also to help you unravel after a long day at work. You can also use it whenever you find yourself feeling tired and stressed – whatever the time of day.

Simple stretch routine

Take off your shoes. If possible, wear loose, comfortable clothes. Take the stretches slowly and carefully: don't overstretch. The idea is to feel the stretch, but not to cause yourself any discomfort or pain. Don't 'bounce' the stretch to make it more intense: once in the pose, hold it without movement. If you cannot achieve the full stretch, go as far as you can. You will find that, with practice, you swiftly increase your flexibility.

Before you begin, warm up your muscles by marching on the spot, swinging your arms as you walk. You may prefer to dance to the radio. It doesn't matter what you do as long as you warm up before stretching – for at least 5 minutes. Using a mini-trampoline, or rebounder, is a great way to warm up – and it will wake up your lymphatic system, too.

1 **CALF STRETCH** Facing a wall, stand a little distance away and, crossing your arms, lean them against the wall. Now lean your forehead against your hands. Bend your left knee and extend your right leg out behind you. Keep both feet parallel, pointing straight ahead. Slowly move your hips forwards, keeping your feet flat, until you feel a slight stretch in the calf muscles of the extended leg. Hold gently for a slow count of ten. Now change legs and repeat.
2 **QUADRICEPS AND KNEE STRETCH** Keeping your right hand on the wall for support, reach behind your back with your left hand and grasp your right foot by the toes. Keep your supporting knee softly bent; tuck your pelvis forwards and stand up straight. Hold gently for a count of 20 and release. Now do the same with the other hand and foot.
3 **GROIN STRETCH** Sit on the floor with the soles of your feet together. Put your hands on your feet and pull your heels in towards your body. This is a strong stretch, so don't worry if you can't get very far at first. Now gently pull your body forwards, towards your feet, keeping your back erect until you feel a stretch. Hold for a count of 20. As you hold the stretch, concentrate on relaxing your arms, shoulders and feet.

4 HAMSTRING STRETCH Still sitting, straighten your left leg out in front of you. Keep your right leg bent as in the groin stretch, but now bring the sole of the foot to face the inside of the outstretched leg (as far as you can). Keep the extended leg slightly bent. Now bend forwards slightly, from the hips, with your hands relaxed on the floor next to the extended leg, until you feel an easy stretch. Touch the top of the thigh of your left leg and check it is feeling soft and relaxed. Keep the foot of your extended leg upright, not turned out. Hold for a count of 30. Now release the stretch and repeat with your right leg extended.

5 UPPER HAMSTRINGS AND HIP STRETCH With your left leg extended in front of you, bend your right leg and bring it up towards your abdomen, cradling it in your arms like a baby. Gently pull the leg towards you until you feel an easy stretch. Hold for a count of 20, release and then repeat with the other leg.

6 ARCH STRETCH Sit on your toes (kneeling, but so you are resting your buttocks on your heels with your toes on the floor). Keep your hands on the floor in front of you for balance. Gently stretch the arches of the feet. Hold for a count of ten.

7 ARM STRETCH Bring yourself gently to your feet. Raise your left arm above your head. Grasp it at the elbow with your right hand. Now, let your left hand drop down behind your shoulder blade (or as far as it can go). Gently pull the left arm back and in towards the head. Keep your arm, neck and shoulders relaxed. Hold for a count of 20, then release and repeat on the other side.

8 ALL-OVER STRETCH Stand upright with your feet shoulder-width apart, feet facing forwards. Extend your arms in front of you at chest height with palms touching. Now separate them bring them slowly back and down, then on behind your back. Clasp your hands behind your back with your arms extended straight down (hands level with your buttocks). Now inhale deeply, pulling your shoulders back. Exhale and bend forwards, raising your arms (still clasped at the hands) over your head. Return very slowly to an upright position with your arms held loosely behind your back with hands clasped. Slowly twist to the right and then to the left. Repeat the whole stretch three times.

9 BACK STRETCH Sit down and bring your knees up to your chest (with your ankles crossed). Clasp your knees with both arms. Drop your head down to your knees and roll backwards on your spine. Roll forwards and backwards several times.

10 SPINE STRETCH Lie down on the floor. Lift your pelvis slightly and then release. Bend your knees and slowly let them twist over to the right. Turn your head to the left and press your shoulders into the floor. Hold for a few minutes, then bring your knees back to centre and repeat on the other side.

Yoga

Yoga is a wonderful form of exercise for absolutely everyone. It has myriad benefits. It puts health-giving pressure on all the body's organs and muscles systematically. It tones the liver, lungs, kidneys, spleen, intestines and heart. The precise postures of yoga (known as asanas) cause the blood to circulate more freely, nourishing your organs and softening muscle and ligament tissue. Deep stretching brings the skeletal, fascial and muscular systems back into alignment; it also lubricates the joints, making you far more flexible.

Yoga is used to ease bad backs, to help heal asthma and for breathing difficulties. It can be a splendid exercise both during and after pregnancy. Some yoga teachers run special classes for new mothers to which they can take (and include) their babies! However, do ensure that your yoga teacher is properly qualified (usually the term yoga therapist conveys this) to handle medical conditions.

Yoga helps to detoxify the body – and also the mind. When you practise yoga, your nervous system shifts into 'relax' mode, switching from the sympathetic to the para-sympathetic nervous system, so you feel calm, cool and in control.

Cautions

- If you are a beginner, always go to a qualified teacher, rather than trying to teach yourself from a book or video.
- Find a well-qualified teacher. If you have any health problems (particularly a heart condition, back trouble or if you have had any kind of surgery), you should find a yoga therapist (who has had a strict medical training), rather than a yoga teacher.
- Don't push yourself beyond your limits. Yoga is not competitive – everyone works at his or her own pace and within the body's limits. Start small – you will soon find you can stretch further or work harder.
- Make sure your yoga teacher is aware of any health or fitness problems you have before the class. A good teacher will be able to tell you which postures to avoid and will often give you specific postures to help your condition.
- If you are pregnant, you will need to avoid certain postures. Again, you should see a yoga therapist or find a class specifically designed for pregnant women.

The Sun Salute – a complete workout for body, mind and spirit

The Sun Salute or Salutation to the Sun is a well-known yoga routine. It is perhaps the most effective series of exercises you can do for your body. In ancient India, the Sun Salute was a part of daily spiritual practice and was performed in the very early morning facing the sun, the deity for health and longevity. If you are feeling very keen, follow this practice and greet the dawn with this series of exercises. Otherwise, perform them on rising, facing east.

There are 12 spinal positions and each stretches different ligaments and moves the spine in different ways. At first, this series of exercises will seem jerky and uncoordinated, but persevere. As you begin to learn the positions off by heart, you will find you can move fluidly and smoothly from one to another. Start off with just one whole set and gradually build up to the optimum 12. You may find it helpful to record the instructions on a tape recorder until you become familiar enough with them to do without.

1 Standing upright, bring your feet together so that your big toes are touching. Your arms are by your sides. Relax your shoulders and tuck your chin in slightly – look straight ahead, not down at your feet. Bring your hands together in front of your chest with palms together, as if you were praying. Exhale deeply.

2 Inhale slowly and deeply while you bring your arms straight up over your head, placing your palms together as you finish inhaling. Look gently backwards towards your thumbs. Lift the knees by tightening your thighs. Reach up as far as possible, lengthening your whole body. If you feel comfortable, you can take the posture back slightly further into a bend.

3 Exhale as you bend forwards, so that your hands are in line with your feet. Your head should be touching your knees. To begin with, you might find you have to bend your knees in order to reach the floor. Eventually, with practice, you should be able to straighten your knees into the full posture.

4 Inhale deeply and move your left leg away from your body in a large backward sweep, so that you end up in a kind of extended lunge position. Make sure that you keep your hands and right foot firmly on the ground. Your right knee should be positioned between your hands. Now bend your head upwards, stretching out your back.

5 Exhaling deeply, bring yourself into an arched position. Your arms are in front of your head, palms facing directly in front, arms shoulder-width apart. Your back should be in a straight line, with your head in line with your arms. Keep your feet and heels flat on the floor.

6 Exhale and lower your body onto the floor. This is a curious posture known as *sastanga namaskar,* or the eight-curved prostration, because only eight parts of

your body should be in contact with the floor: your feet, your knees, your hands, your chest and your forehead. Try to keep your abdomen raised and, if you can possibly manage it, keep your nose off the floor so only your forehead makes contact. Don't worry if it's an impossibility at this point – just keep the idea in mind.

7 Inhale deeply and bend up into the position known as the cobra – hands on the floor in front of you, arms straight, bending backwards as far as feels comfortable. Look upwards.

8 Exhale deeply and lift your back into position 5 (known as the dog). Remember to keep your feet and heels (if you can) flat on the floor. Once again, with regular practice, you will find that this becomes easier.

9 Inhale deeply and return to posture 4, this time with the opposite leg forwards, so that your left foot is in line with your hands, while your right leg is stretched back.

10 Exhale deeply and return to posture 3.

11 Raise the arms overhead and bend backwards as you inhale (as for posture 2).

12 Return to a comfortable standing position, feet together, with your arms by your sides. Look straight ahead and exhale. To close, bring your hands back together in a position of prayer.

Further yoga postures for health and vitality

As you become more proficient in yoga, you can extend your practice. Once you have performed your sun salutations, you may like to include these postures, all of which will help to increase energy and eliminate toxins. Perform them slowly and carefully in a controlled manner. Never race. If you feel any pain, stop doing that exercise. You should just feel a gentle stretch.

PRAYER POSTURE
This gentle posture puts all your internal organs into balance. It encourages deep breathing and helps to align your spine into its optimum position. It is also deeply calming for the mind.

1 Stand with your feet together and parallel. Aim to stand tall without straining – imagine you have a string connecting your head to the ceiling.

2 Check your head – it should be easily balanced on your neck, with eyes gazing softly ahead. Your chin should be neither tucked in nor jutting out.

3 Tilt your pelvis slightly forwards and keep your knees straight, but soft – don't lock them.

4 Now bring your hands palms together in front of your chest, as if you were praying.

5 Relax your jaw, your facial muscles and your shoulders. Breathe softly and regularly. You may want to focus lightly on an object in front of you, or you can gently close your eyes.

6 Hold this pose for a few minutes or for as long as you feel comfortable. Then bring your hands back down to your sides and resume your normal stance.

THE TREE
This is a classic yoga posture which is superb for improving your balance, concentration and coordination.

1 Stand up tall and straight. Your feet should be close together and parallel. Fix your eyes gently on something (you will need to keep your eyes open for this posture), and breathe naturally and regularly.

2 Lift one leg and place the sole of your foot against the inner side of your other thigh. You can use your hands to place it there. Keep focusing on the point ahead of you.

3 Now bring your hands up into a prayer position in front of your chest.

4 Hold the posture for as long as feels comfortable. Focus on your breathing. Think about the strength and poise of a tree – its roots firm in the ground, its branches reaching towards heaven.

5 Rest for a few moments before repeating the posture with the other leg.

CHILD POSTURE

This looks very simple, but has very deep effects. It massages your internal organs, promoting good circulation and aiding elimination. It also helps to keep your spine supple and flexible.

1 Kneel down, keeping your legs pressed together. Lower your buttocks so that you are sitting on your heels.

2 Now bend forwards slowly until your forehead is resting on the floor. You may not be able to get this far, but don't worry, just go as far as is comfortable. If it helps, you can rest your head on a cushion.

3 Bring your arms behind you so your hands rest on the floor next to your feet. Relax.

4 Stay in this posture for as long as you feel comfortable. Try to keep your breathing regular and relaxed.

THE MOUNTAIN

This seated variation of the mountain posture tones your abdominal muscles and improves your breathing. It can help sluggish circulation and can also tone the muscles in the back.

1 Sit cross-legged on the floor. Hold yourself upright and breathe naturally and easily.

2 Inhale and stretch your arms up over your head to form a steeple shape over your head. Keep the insides of your arms close to your ears. Bring your palms together if you can and press them together as if you were praying.

3 Hold this posture for as long as you can comfortably do so. Remember to breathe easily and regularly as you hold the pose.

4 Exhale and slowly lower your arms to your lap. Rest for a few moments and then repeat.

Chi kung – simple but effective

Chi kung (also known as qi gong) is another marvellous form of mind–body exercise. It combines breathing techniques with precise movements and mental concentration. If you practise chi kung regularly, you will reap myriad benefits; your energy levels will increase, while your stress levels fall. Practitioners say you might also prevent or cure any number of chronic or acute diseases. Chi kung is said to improve concentration and even increase creativity and inspiration.

Best of all, absolutely anyone can do chi kung. If you are too weak to stand, there are sitting exercises. If you can't even sit, there are lying-down exercises! Chi kung has helped people in wheelchairs and those recovering from illness and injury – even the very elderly can benefit.

Don't think, however, that because chi kung exercises look simple, they are consequently easy. Chi kung is a precise discipline, demanding meticulous concentration and patience. It is also surprisingly tough on the muscles.

Ideally, you should strive to practise chi kung every day, even if only for 5 or 10 minutes. You can try the following exercises to start with. Wear loose, comfortable clothing and keep your feet bare.

The starting posture

This is the basic starting posture of chi kung. It puts you in the correct position and helps you to become aware of your entire body.

1　Stand with your feet shoulder-width apart. Make sure you find your natural balance – your weight should be neither too far forwards nor too far back, or it will lead to tension and tiredness.

2　Feel the rim of your foot, your heel, your little toe and big toe relaxed on the ground.

3　Keep your knees relaxed. Check to ensure that your knees are exactly over your feet.

4　Relax your lower back. Relax your stomach and buttocks.

5　Let your chest become hollow. Relax and slightly round your shoulders.

6　Imagine you have a pigtail on top of your head that is tied to a rafter on the roof. Let your head float lightly and freely. Relax your tongue, mouth and jaw.

7　Stay in this position for a few moments, with your hands hanging loosely by your sides.

8　Now spend some time visualizing the five elements of Chinese philosophy. Start with earth (imagine the feeling of weight and rootedness); then water (looseness and fluidity); air (lightness and transparency); fire (sparkle – remember this should be fun!); and space (envisage the space within each joint, muscle, breath and your mind).

9　Throughout your chi kung practice, keep bringing your mind gently back to your posture – this will help to keep your mind restful.

Holding the dantien

This exercise stimulates the dantien, which in chi kung is considered to be the storehouse of chi or qi, the body's vital energy. It is also good for circulation and lymph drainage, and helps to promote deep, effective breathing. The dantien is located about an inch or so below the navel.

1　Stand in the starting position.

2　Men should place their left hand on the dantien, and then the right hand over the left. Women should place their right hand on the dantien, with the left hand over it. Relax your whole body and lightly concentrate your thoughts on the dantien.

3　With the legs straight but not locked, breathe into the dantien. You will feel your abdomen inflate under your hands as you do this.

4　Slowly bend your knees and breathe out. Your abdomen will deflate into the body on the out breath. Repeat this exercise for at least two minutes – as you get more used to it, you can continue it for longer.

Supporting the sky

This exercise is excellent for the lungs and breathing – it is superb when performed first thing in the morning because it empties the lungs after sleeping. It's also very helpful if you have backache. Incidentally, it could be very beneficial if you suffer from repetitive strain injury (RSI).

1　Stand in the starting position.

2　Hold your hands in front of your dantien so the palms face up and the fingers point to each other.

3　Raise your hands up past the front of your chest, with the palms now facing the body. Breathe in. As your hands come up, keep your back straight and, when the hands reach the face, roll your hands over (so that the palms face upwards). Stretch your arms up and look upwards.

4　Open your arms out to the sides and lower them while bending the knees. Keep the back straight until the hands are in the starting position, but now with your knees bent. Breathe out at the same time. Repeat at least five or six times for the maximum benefit.

Turning the head and twisting the tail

This exercise helps to get the kidneys working well, so that they can efficiently eliminate toxins. It strengthens the spine and helps keep it flexible and strong. It takes a fair bit of coordination, but do persist, as it is highly effective.

1 Stand in the chi kung starting position, but with the arms held out and raised at the sides of the body to shoulder height.
2 Place your weight on the right leg, keeping both legs relaxed. Lean to the left while raising your right arm slightly. Allow the left arm to curve downwards, so the tips of your fingers touch your left thigh about where a trouser seam would be. Turn your head to look into the palm of the right hand. As you perform this move, exhale.
3 Come back to the starting position with your arms held out and raised at the sides, breathing in as you do so.
4 Now shift your weight onto the left leg and lean to the right, raising your left arm slightly and curving the right arm downwards, so the fingertips touch the right thigh. Turn your head to look into the palm of the right hand. Breathe out as you perform this move.
5 Repeat at least five times for each side, keeping your movements slow and flowing.

Dragon stamping

This exercise is great for your circulation and balance, both mental and physical. It helps to calm the mind and, if performed in the morning, helps you to become focused and energized for the day ahead. Make sure that you are breathing out as you rise and in as you return – it's easy to get it the wrong way round, which is far less effective.

1 Stand in the starting position.
2 While breathing out, rise slowly onto your tiptoes, as high as you can. Stretch your body upwards through the back, keeping the abdomen relaxed. At the same time, point your fingers down and inwards, stretching your arms downwards as you do so.
3 Return your heels slowly to the ground on the in breath and relax. Repeat at least five times.

Breathing

We take breathing for granted. We all know how to do it and, because we are doing it all the time, we tend to forget about it. However, if you truly want to improve your health, there is no escaping the need for good breathing. Even if you do nothing else for your health, simply taking the time and trouble to learn how to breathe in the optimum way can deliver truly amazing benefits for you, body, mind and spirit.

Why? Because, quite simply, breathing is the way we pull in oxygen and circulate it around the body to 'feed' each and every cell. Equally, breathing is the way we push out carbon dioxide and waste products, 'cleaning out' each and every cell. You simply can't overdose on deep good breathing – the more oxygen you can send around your body, the better. The more effectively you can clear waste from your body, the better. Practitioners of Eastern practices such as yoga and chi kung say that breathing fully can do everything from improving your moods to increasing your resistance to colds and illness, fostering better sleep and even minimize the effects of ageing. It feeds the brain, calms the nerves and has a measurable effect on a number of medical conditions, lowering heart rate and metabolic rate, normalizing blood pressure and decreasing the risks of cardiovascular disease.

So what's wrong with our breathing? Basically, we nearly all breathe too shallowly, almost cautiously, only using a tiny portion of our lungs. It has been estimated that, when we breathe in, we take in only around a tumblerful of air when we could, in fact, take in at least three times that amount. Why do we need to take in more air? Because the lungs are made up of some 700 million air sacs, of which the greater proportion lie in the lower lungs. When we breathe shallowly, we don't ever wholly expel all the waste gases and detritus in the lower lungs. We also run the risk of losing vital elasticity in the lower part of our lungs. On a more esoteric level, good breathing techniques transport vital energy (qi, chi or prana) right around the body. As you become more proficient, you can boost the power of your breathing by visualizing health-giving energy flooding into your lungs and thence to your entire body as you inhale and stale, spent energy pouring out as you exhale. In China, it is said that breathing like this will enliven your metabolism and invigorate all the cells of your body, producing good health and long life.

Fortunately, there are very simple exercises that can help bring our breathing back to its optimum fullness and freedom. The yogic tradition in India developed a whole science of good breathing. They called it *pranayama*, the art of breath control and expansion. In China, the effects of the breathing that forms an integral part of the chi kung (or qi gong) exercises have been rigorously tested. Hospitals have cured patients of tuberculosis using solely chi kung. Experiments have also shown that chi kung exercises can increase lung capacity from an average of 428.5 cc to 561.8 cc. While the patients were performing the exercises, their lung capacity expanded right up to 1,167.8 cc. Their breathing rate calmed and dropped, and their brainwaves dropped into the theta level, allowing the patients to remain alert, yet deeply calm.

The average person breathes around 16 times a minute, while a chi kung practitioner, through practice, breathes slowly and deeply just five or six times a minute. Once you start breathing properly, you should notice changes in your entire life. Some people say that how you breathe is a good indication of how you look at life as a whole. Symbolically, breathing is all about taking in the new and eliminating the old.

The Buddhist traditions regard every new breath as giving new life and every exhalation as a little death. Taking in deep, joyful breaths is seen as a way of affirming life and vitality. Breathing minimally and shallowly is turning your back on life or accepting it only grudgingly. As one proverb states: 'Life is in the breath. Therefore, he who only half breathes, half lives.'

Ayurvedic breathing

John Douillard, a trainer who uses ayurvedic principles in his work, teaches all his students to breathe through the nose at all times. This may seem strange if you are used to gasping in huge gulps of air, but Douillard insists that this is the only way to enable the body to enjoy the benefits of exercise without overstretching or stressing it. His 'Darth Vader' breath is a form of pranayama (see below) called *ujjayi* or the 'victorious' breath. This form of breathing is also taught if you take up ashtanga or power yoga. In fact, it is nigh-on impossible to practice ashtanga without it.

• Breathe in through the nose.
• Breathe out through the nose, slightly constricting the throat so you make a guttural sound – like Darth Vader in *Star Wars*. You will feel a sensation in your throat, rather than your nose.
• Notice that your stomach muscles slightly contract as you breathe out.

You will find at first that, breathing in this way, you can work for far less time. Don't panic. Just slow down your workout to suit your breath and your body. You will quickly find that, breathing in this way, you will be able to return to your former fitness levels – and even surpass them.

Simple techniques for better breathing

CHI KUNG – THE ABDOMINAL BREATH
1 Stand with your feet about shoulder-width apart, your knees slightly bent. Relax your shoulders. Imagine that a string runs from the top of your head to the

ceiling, holding you upright but not rigid. Place your hands gently over your stomach, just below your navel.

2 Take in a slow, steady breath through your nose, allowing your abdomen to swell out like a balloon as you breathe. Hold the breath gently.

3 Exhale, allowing the breath to come out slowly through your mouth as the stomach subsides.

This form of breathing directs qi, or vital energy, right around the body. As you become more proficient, imagine health-giving energy flooding into your lungs as you breathe in and stale, spent energy pouring out as you exhale. Apparently, regular practice improves not only your health, but also your beauty!

PRANAYAMA – THE BREATH OF LIFE

1 Lie down on the floor and make yourself comfortable. Bring your feet close to your buttocks and let the feet fall apart, bringing the soles of the feet together, hands resting gently on the floor. (This may feel uncomfortable. If so, you can put cushions under your knees.) This posture stretches the lower abdomen, which enhances the breathing process.

2 Breathe down into the diaphragm, feeling the abdomen expand and contract. Breathe naturally at your own pace, pausing for a second or two between each breath.

3 Now extend the breath so it comes up from the abdomen into the chest. Continue this cycle, pausing slightly between each breath.

4 Finally, bring your knees together and gently stretch out the legs. Allow yourself to relax comfortably on the ground for a few minutes. (You may feel more comfortable with a cushion under your lower back or your neck.)

CAUTION: anyone with chest problems should take these exercises very slowly and carefully, preferably under the guidance of a trained yoga therapist. Anyone with a heart condition, blood pressure problems or glaucoma should not hold the breath. Again, consult a trained yoga therapist.

11 Posture

When thinking about ways to improve our wellbeing, our posture doesn't usually come to mind. Yet we could all feel a lot better in body, mind and spirit if we paid a little more attention to our poise.

As young children, if we were lucky, we possessed unselfconscious poise and perfect posture. We were ideally balanced and fluid. But, as time and modern living take their toll, we tend to adapt ourselves to a harsh environment and a stressful life. We begin to lose our easy freedom of movement when we start adapting to our environment – sitting in badly designed chairs, spending hours at the wheels of our cars, facing difficult emotional trials and traumas. We unconsciously acquire patterns of movement that work against our bodies' design and, in so doing, build up tension.

Long-term tension and bad posture can set us up for back pain and more. The ribs are attached to the upper (thoracic) spine and, when we stoop or round our shoulders, the lungs are not able to expand properly. With long-term misuse, respiratory problems can occur. Habitual slumping in an (albeit comfortable) armchair puts pressure on all your internal organs. Your heart, digestion, lungs and so on are all squeezed and therefore cannot work as effectively as they should. Inevitably, slouching can cause problems if continued on a long-term basis.

Basic good posture involves having your body in the best possible alignment: with back and abdominal muscles equally strong and the spine in the optimum position. Good posture will help your body operate more effectively, but can even affect your mood as well. All the nerve pathways that leave the brain eventually go through muscles, so there is a definite connection between what we think and what we experience. People with an upright posture tend to be confident and extrovert, while those who slump and slouch may veer towards depression and uncertainty. Turning that around has interesting effects. If you are feeling down and depressed, try sitting up straight with your eyes looking ahead – you'll find it automatically lifts your mood.

Good posture – the basic rules

STANDING
- Stand straight: think about standing on both feet. This may sound strange, but most people actually slouch to one side, putting their weight on one leg, which puts them out of balance. Study the basic posture of chi kung (page 78), which will put you in a good standing position.
- Practise the pelvic tilt: tuck your bottom in and pull your stomach in so that you are using your muscles almost like a girdle to hold yourself in. This provides good support for the lower back.
- Bring your chin in: most of us poke our chins out far too far. The head should be balanced, with the chin tucked in.

WALKING
- Take even strides: some people pull themselves along, overusing their hamstrings (the back of the thighs); others lean forwards and overstride. The healthiest way to walk is to take even strides.
- Keep your balance: we are designed to balance on one leg after the other. Don't throw your weight around.
- Walk low: high heels can throw the pelvis forwards which, in turn, will throw the whole body out of alignment. This will eventually cause shortening in some muscles, which could lead to back pain. Low, well-cushioned shoes are best for everyday wear. It's fine to wear high heels for special occasions – just don't wear them all day, every day.

SITTING – FOR WORK
- Chair comfort: you should be seated with your knees lower than your pelvis. The seat should be high enough for you to relax your shoulders, leaving your arms at a 90-degree angle to your desk. If the chair has arms, they should be low enough to fit under your desk.
- Screen daze: if you use a screen at work, your computer should be on a stand, rather than on the desk, so that you can look directly at it, rather than down towards it. Equally, make sure it is placed directly in front of you, rather than off to one side.

SITTING – TO RELAX
- Don't slump: slumping in front of the television may feel comfortable, but it's the worst possible position for your back. You should have a reasonably firm support behind you – a firm cushion will help.
- Watch your eyes: if you're watching television, you should be directly facing it with your head balanced. Don't twist. If you're reading a book or magazine, lift it up towards you, rather than bending over your lap.

SLEEPING
- Get the right support: a good mattress is essential. Too soft and the curves of your back sink in and reinforce bad posture – but, equally, too hard can be uncomfortable.
- Choose your pillow carefully: it needs to be malleable enough to mould to the curves of your neck. There are specialist pillows available on the market that ensure this, or you could roll up a hand towel and place it inside your pillowcase to provide a good support for your neck.
- Lie well: it's fine to sleep on either your side or your back, but avoid sleeping on your front with your head to one side. It twists the upper neck and can create imbalance.

WHAT TO AVOID
Certain movements and practices will play havoc with your posture – and your health. These are the main ones to avoid.
1. The heavy shoulder bag: a shoulder bag actually pulls up the shoulder, causing your body to overbalance and twist to compensate. A rucksack is ideal or, at the very least, keep shifting sides when carrying heavy bags.
2. The telephone shrug: clutching the telephone between ear and shoulder may result in 'telephone neck syndrome', which can cause searing pain between the shoulder blades. If you spend most of your day telephoning, use a headset.
3. The reversing rick: when reversing a car, don't pull your head back sharply and jerk your neck around. Instead, try dropping the tip of your nose towards your shoulder and then turning it while imagining your shoulder lengthening.
4. Post-exercise trauma: good posture after vigorous sport is very important. Don't slump in the changing room. Stand up and walk about instead.
5. The hip bend: bever pick up anything by twisting and bending – always squat before lifting.

Alexander technique

A straightforward, down-to-earth technique could make you taller and slimmer. It can see off silence stress and banish the blues. It can even give significant relief from back and neck pain and the ache of arthritis. Yet this technique is no new wonder therapy, no esoteric healing – it's been taught for years. It's called the Alexander technique.

It was developed by Frederick Mathias Alexander, an Australian born in 1869. Alexander was a successful actor – until he started to lose his voice during orations. A host of doctors and voice coaches could find nothing wrong with him, so Alexander reasoned that he was doing something during his performance to cause the problem. With the use of a series of mirrors, he analysed his movements and discovered he was pulling his head back and down onto his spine with an enormous amount of tension. The tension was impairing his breathing and causing constriction of the larynx.

Alexander began to experiment and finally came up with a solution for the tension. He gave his body three main orders: 'Allow the neck to be free'; 'Allow the neck to go forwards and upwards'; and 'Allow the back to lengthen and widen.' These mental instructions both relaxed the tension and freed his voice. In addition, he discovered that the asthma he had suffered from since birth also vanished.

Alexander was so intrigued by these findings that he developed an entire system that would enable almost anyone to regain the comfort and ease of movement they enjoyed as babies and small children.

Our bodies will cope with postural abuses for some time, but then, generally from our thirties on, they start to complain. We begin to develop neck and back pains; we start getting headaches or migraines; we feel permanently tense and stressed, and have trouble sleeping. Some of us develop breathing problems because our lungs are cramped; others suffer digestive problems because we are squashing our colons. The Alexander technique offers us a solution, teaching us how to unravel taut, tense bodies.

The Alexander technique may not be exciting or trendy, but it does work. And, once you have learnt the technique, it is yours for life – along with all the benefits of a body that is deeply relaxed and comfortable in itself.

What can the Alexander technique help?

- Alexander technique teachers don't claim to help or cure anything, but do say that it is almost always therapeutic.
- Many people (especially those with neck and back pain, and arthritis) are referred by their doctors.
- Many psychologists find that the Alexander technique can often help to clear depression. There seems to be a strong link between posture and psychological problems. Simply 'straightening up' and looking the world in the eye appears to have an instant effect on mood.
- Arthritis seems to respond well.
- Some people with asthma find they breathe more easily after learning the Alexander technique.
- It improves coordination and flexibility.
- Its pupils regularly report that they feel easier in themselves, that they have more energy and less stress.
- Many people 'grow' (in fact, they are actually straightening up) by as much as 3 or 4 cm (an inch and a half) after learning the Alexander technique, and they also appear to lose weight. We have a tendency to sink into our hips, so therefore, by encouraging a lengthening of the torso, a redistribution of fat tissue takes place and the body becomes taller and thinner.

What can I expect from a session?

WHERE WILL I HAVE THE TREATMENT?
You will be in the teacher's room.

WILL I BE CLOTHED?
Yes, you remain fully clothed throughout.

WHAT HAPPENS?
The technique is usually taught in individual lessons or small classes. Your teacher will meticulously observe how you use your body when you are standing, sitting and walking. He or she will then teach you how to change your patterns of movement subtly to restore your body to its natural balance. Don't expect miracles overnight – a basic course will consist of around 30 lessons and many people go on to take still more.

WILL IT HURT?
No, it's not painful at all.

WILL ANYTHING STRANGE HAPPEN?
No, not really. The exercises are all pretty straightforward.

WILL I BE GIVEN ANYTHING TO TAKE?
No, medication is not part of the treatment.

IS THERE ANY HOMEWORK?
Yes, lots. You will be expected to put everything you learn in the lessons into practice.

Do-it-yourself Alexander technique – relieving tension

This simple Alexander exercise can help relieve muscular tension. It involves lying on the floor with your head supported by a small pile of books. The number of books you will need will depend on your height and the curvature of your spine. Stand normally with your heels, buttocks and shoulder blades lightly touching a wall. Get a friend to measure the distance between your head and the wall, and add about 2½ cm (1 in) to the measurement – this is the height of books you will need. Choose paperbacks (they're much more comfortable!).

- Lie on your back on the floor by going on all fours, then gently rolling onto the books. Bring your feet as near to your buttocks as is comfortable, so your knees point to the ceiling. Your hands should gently rest on either side of your navel.
- Lie like this for about 20 minutes. During this time, try to become aware of any tension in your body. Is your back arched so it is not fully in contact with the ground? Are your shoulders hunched? Are your shoulder blades not fully in contact with the ground? Do the books feel hard because you are pulling your head back, causing tension in your neck? Can you feel one side of your body more in contact with the floor than the other? Can you feel tension in your legs – do they want to fall in or out to the sides? Can you feel more pressure on the outside or the inside of your feet?
- Don't move or try to correct any problems – that will only make them worse. Instead, apply conscious thought to help release tension. If your back is arched, think of it lengthening and widening. If your shoulders are hunched, imagine them dropping away from your ears. If your leg wants to fall out, think of your knees pointing up to the ceiling.
- Before getting up from the floor, pause for a moment – think about a less stressful way of rising to your feet. Roll over onto your stomach and go on all fours. Assume a kneeling position and then put one foot in front of the other to come back up to a standing position.

Feldenkrais method

The Feldenkrais method has been described as a way to 'find the cat in you' – teaching effortless movement through improved mind and body coordination. It's the secret behind the poise and control of countless actors and dancers, and the magic ingredient that can give sportspeople the edge in improving their performance or fine-tuning their game.

The Feldenkrais method was developed by Moshe Feldenkrais, who was born in Russia in 1904 and gained a PhD in engineering and physics. When he damaged his knee playing football, he was told that the only treatment was (possibly ineffectual) surgery. Feldenkrais decided to tackle the problem himself, applying his knowledge of structure and motion, combined with his martial-arts training.

He concluded that stiffness and pain are often caused not by physical defects, disease and degeneration, but rather by limitations in movement. Re-educating his body to move more freely and easily, he cured his knee and began a quest to help other people find the same release. By gently moving their bodies in unfamiliar ways, Feldenkrais found his 'students' could become more aware of how their bodies moved and, by repeating the actions, could actually alter the neuromuscular patterns that organize and control movement. The result was freedom from pain, increased flexibility and a wonderful feeling of truly inhabiting the body.

Feldenkrais is often compared to the Alexander technique, and the two systems certainly share the same emphasis of educating the body into freedom of posture and movement. However, whereas Alexander seeks the ideal, for perfect posture, Feldenkrais will be happy with a simple improvement on what you already have.

What can the Feldenkrais method help?

- Physiotherapists often refer clients to Feldenkrais teachers for help in easing pain, chronic back problems and neuromuscular diseases.
- It can help people recover from accidents and strokes.
- It's a wonderful destresser – particularly for people who spend a lot of time in front of a computer.
- It can help minimize the severity of repetitive strain injury (RSI).
- 'Clumsy' children can benefit.
- Elderly people find it helps them move with added freedom.
- It gives flexibility, strength and suppleness, which, in turn, makes people feel more confident.

What can I expect from a session?

WHERE WILL I HAVE THE TREATMENT?
You will be in the teacher's room on a couch, or in a hall if you are being taught in a class.

WILL I BE CLOTHED?
Yes, you stay fully clothed throughout.

WHAT HAPPENS?
The Feldenkrais method is taught in two distinct ways. One-to-one sessions are known as Functional Integration and comprise manipulation, generally carried out on a low couch. It's all very gentle, minimal and pleasant. You will be asked often to 'check in' with your body, noticing sensations and getting in touch with how you feel. You will also be taught how to perform the minute movements for yourself. A lot of visualization is involved, to help your body make the right moves. There is no pulling or straining; everything is done slowly, carefully and mindfully. You can also learn the method in Awareness

through Movement classes and workshops, in which small groups carry out gentle exercises guided by a teacher. Many of the movements taught in class are drawn directly from babyhood and childhood, so you're quite likely to find yourself rolling or twisting on the floor just like a toddler. Great fun!

WILL IT HURT?
No. You may notice some clicks and pops, but it's very pleasant and soothing.

WILL ANYTHING STRANGE HAPPEN?
Often you will be asked to compare the two sides of your body, halfway through the session. You may be surprised to find that the side that has been worked on will feel quite different from the one that hasn't.

WILL I BE GIVEN ANYTHING TO TAKE?
No, medication is not part of the treatment.

IS THERE ANY HOMEWORK?
Yes, you will be expected to practise at home what you learn in sessions or classes.

Mézières method

The Mézières method teaches that perfection is possible. Within us all lies the potential to become 'a Greek god or goddess': no saddlebag thighs, no bulging bottoms, no rounded shoulders, no flabby waists. It isn't merely a fantasy: this unique form of bodywork really can resculpt the body. By returning your body to its ideal form, you will automatically bring yourself to a better state of health.

The method is well respected in its native France, where it has been quietly revolutionizing bodywork for the past 40 years. Its originator was Françoise Mézières, a teacher of physiotherapy and anatomy. Like all physiotherapists, she had been taught that the muscles in the back are generally too weak and need to be strengthened. But one day, while examining a patient, it suddenly struck her that in fact the very opposite was true: the muscles in the back were actually too strong. Their strength caused them to become shortened and to lose their elasticity, creating tension and eventually pain. This imbalance of muscle strength was occurring all over the body, but it was particularly pronounced in the back because the muscles in the back overlapped to form a chain running the entire length of the body.

There was, she realized, absolutely no point in relieving stiffness or shortening in just one muscle or muscle group, as it would simply cause compensatory shortening in another area: the whole chain needed to be stretched and readjusted at the same time. This concept flatly contradicted everything Mézières believed in, everything she taught her students, so she set out to disprove her theory. Two years later, after constant observation and evaluation, she admitted defeat and began to reshape entirely her way of working.

The Mézières method is no easy ride. It involves intense, painstaking work by practitioner *and* patient. Expect to have sessions once or twice a week and for it to take several months, possibly a year, to reshape a body. Practitioners say you can often get rid of pain in one session, but it will never be long-lasting unless you work hard to correct the cause of that pain. This correction involves literally unravelling the distortions of the body – it's a little like slowly and patiently taking the kinks and knots out of a badly twisted rope and stretching it so that it once again it lies smooth and flat.

What can the Mézières method help?

- People report a radical reshaping of their bodies after using the Mézières method.
- Aches and pains often disappear with this therapy; so, too, can arthritis and sciatica.

- The Mézières method can correct long-term distortions of the body, from kyphosis (dowager's hump) and scoliosis (spinal curvature) to flat feet, knock knees and bow legs.
- It has a positive effect on mood as well, improving confidence, easing depression and soothing anxiety.
- Practitioners promise that the Mézières method can correct almost any problem, bar those that are congenital or caused by fractures or mutilations.

What can I expect from a session?

WHERE WILL I HAVE THE TREATMENT?
You will be lying on the floor in the therapist's room.

WILL I BE CLOTHED?
You will be asked to strip down to underwear.

WHAT HAPPENS?
First, the practitioner gauges your posture, asking you to stand with feet together, ankles, knees and toes touching, then to bend forwards slowly as if to touch your toes. You will be observed from all angles, as the practitioner decides how to proceed.

You will then lie on the floor while the practitioner puts your body into precise positions. It sounds simple, but it's tough work. You feel rather like an overpacked case: press on one side and something pops out the other side. The practitioner may use his or her body weight to maximize to the stretch, sometimes kneading tense, stiff muscles to help them yield.

WILL IT HURT?
It can be quite uncomfortable at times. You may have pins and needles after the session and it's quite common for your legs to feel numb in the early stages.

WILL ANYTHING STRANGE HAPPEN?
You may well feel totally different after a session, as if you have been given a new body.

WILL I BE GIVEN ANYTHING TO TAKE?
No, medication is not part of the treatment, although some practitioners may advise you on diet.

IS THERE ANY HOMEWORK?
Yes, for best results in reshaping your body, you will practise the Mézières method at home.

Pilates

Pilates has sprung to fame in the past few years. Adored by dancers and sportspeople, it is a gentle exercise system which aims to put you back in touch with your body. The result is perfect poise, fabulous flexibility and freedom from aches and pains.

Pilates was developed more than 60 years ago by Joseph Pilates, a German who was interned in Britain during World War I. He developed a system to maintain the health and fitness levels of himself and his fellow internees while they were in confinement. Later, Pilates moved to New York and his studio became a magnet for ballet dancers, sportspeople, actors and actresses, among many other wise mortals who wanted to learn the workout that gives strength without bulky muscles; the method that promises harmony between your mind and your muscle.

The Pilates method works through resistance – using equipment with tensioned springs, gravity or your own body weight. Pilates is wonderful for correcting any postural imbalances and bad habits, by increasing the mobility, strength and elasticity of your muscles. Considered to be one of the safest forms of exercise ever devised, it is regularly recommended by osteopaths and physiotherapists.

Pilates uses flowing, controlled movements with specific breathing patterns to improve both coordination and muscle stamina. Every movement is carefully monitored to ensure you are using the correct muscles in precisely the correct way.

What can pilates help?

- The Pilates system is invaluable as rehabilitative exercise after injury. It can also help prevent old injuries recurring.
- Pilates is extolled by dancers and sportspeople. Actors, singers and musicians use the method to improve their breath control, grace and coordination.
- It improves posture, relieves back problems and is superb for toning and streamlining the body.
- It is a totally safe form of exercise for use during pregnancy.
- Pilates can help prevent the onset of osteoporosis.
- Stress and stress-related problems respond well.
- It can help repetitive strain injury (RSI).
- The Pilates method is ideal for older people who want to maintain mobility.

What can I expect from a session?

WHERE WILL I HAVE THE SESSION?
You will be in a Pilates studio filled with special equipment – machines, mats, large balls – or a simple room without equipment.

WILL I BE CLOTHED?
Yes, you will wear comfortable clothes for the session. Generally, you will go barefoot.

WHAT HAPPENS?
The teacher will start by finding out about you – your lifestyle, any problems, what you want to achieve. He or she will also check your posture, looking for any imbalances and tension. You will then be taken through a warm-up leading into a series of stretches and exercises. Every movement in Pilates is focused (you will be taught to be mindful of your body throughout) and fluid. You will constantly focus on centring and pulling your stomach muscles in. Every exercise uses the breath in a specific way, as you breathe in through the nose and out through the mouth. These exercises are very precise – because they have been designed to work specific groups of muscles – so expect constant supervision throughout. Often you will perform an exercise in several different ways, with each variation more advanced. However, you will always be advised to work at your own pace and level: nothing is ever pushed in Pilates. Like yoga, it is non-competitive. If you practise regularly, you will soon notice your core strength increasing, allowing you to perform the more advanced variations with ease.

WILL IT HURT?
No, it's not painful. However, you may find some of the exercises quite difficult to begin with.

WILL ANYTHING STRANGE HAPPEN?
No, Pilates is a pretty down-to-earth system.

WILL I BE GIVEN ANYTHING TO TAKE?
No, medication is not part of the system.

IS THERE ANY HOMEWORK?
Yes, for best results, you should not only practise Pilates at home as well, but also as often as possible.

Home Pilates

SLIDING DOWN THE WALL
This releases tension and is great for the spine.
1 Stand with your feet shoulder-width apart and parallel, with your back about 45 cm (18 in) from a wall.
2 Bend your knees and lean back into the wall (as if you were sitting on a stool).
3 Breathe in and feel yourself lengthening up through the spine as the breath fills your lungs.
4 Start to breathe out and gently pull your stomach in, as if you were bringing your belly button back towards the spine.
5 Still breathing out, relax your head and neck so you can let your chin drop forwards. Imagine your forehead has a weight pulling it forwards.
6 Now slowly start to roll forwards. Keep your hands and arms, and your neck and head, relaxed. Make sure your bottom stays glued to the wall. Let yourself roll forwards one vertebra at a time, as if you were being peeled off the wall.
7 Go as far as you feel comfortable (eventually you will be able to reach the floor). Now hang in your furthest position and breathe in.
8 Breathe out and pull your belly button to the spine again. Rotate your pelvis so the pubic bone moves towards your chin (remember these are tiny movements).
9 Slowly, vertebra by vertebra, curl your spine back into the wall as you come up. Repeat this exercise six times.

FOOT CIRCLING
This simple exercise helps keep your ankle joints flexible.
1 Sit on the floor with your legs stretched out in front of you, a little more than shoulder-width apart with your knees facing up to the ceiling. (**NOTE:** if this is uncomfortable, put a pillow under your bottom to tilt you forwards slightly). Place your hands on the floor beside you to balance yourself.
2 Now feel yourself lifting out of your hips, keeping your spine straight.
3 Rotate your feet around in outward circles (your right foot will be going clockwise and your left foot anticlockwise).
4 Keep your knees still and work from your ankles to get a really good range of movement.
5 Repeat with your feet rotating in the opposite (inwards) direction. Repeat the whole exercise ten times.

12 Sleep

Good sleep is vital for our health and happiness. The world seems a brighter place after a good night's slumber. When our sleep is disturbed, on the other hand, nothing seems right. Sleep experts believe that lack of sleep can be blamed for up to 40,000 road crashes a year, for bad decision making in business and even for such disasters as Chernobyl. On a more domestic level, any parent of a poorly sleeping child will tell you that persistent lack of sleep is one of the most exquisite forms of torture ever invented!

But how much sleep do we truly need? Ask the experts and you end up confused. Some say we all suffer from sleep deficit – sleeping, on average, between an hour and 90 minutes less than we should. Others maintain that we need only between 5 or 6 hours, and that most of us are actually oversleeping. So whom should we believe? The answer has to be our own bodies, which undoubtedly know how much sleep we need and when. Most of us will sleep for around 8 hours a night, but some people happily manage on 5 or 6, while others feel lousy without 9. Curiously, our very personalities can determine how much sleep we need. American experts have discovered that short sleepers tend to be efficient, energetic, ambitious people who are relatively sure of themselves, socially adept and decisive. They are satisfied with their lives, while their social and political views are conformist. Long sleepers, by contrast, are nonconformist with mild neurotic problems and tend to be less sure of themselves. They appear to be more artistic or creative.

It's not really how much sleep we get that is important for our health and wellbeing, it is the kind of sleep we get – quality over quantity. Sleep is divided into three types: light, deep and REM (or dreaming) sleep. Cut down on sleep and our bodies will compensate by automatically cutting down first light sleep and then, if necessary, REM sleep, too.

The importance of REM or dreaming sleep is another thorny topic of debate among scientists. Some insist that our dreams are merely the detritus of the day, spewed out like so much garbage. Others are convinced that, by using our dreams creatively, we can resolve many of our waking problems. Many researchers are fascinated by the idea of 'lucid dreaming', of learning how consciously to direct your dreams. Dr Rosalind Cartwright of St Luke's Medical Centre in Chicago found that people who cope best with divorce tend to have helpful dream patterns. She recommends reshaping dreams to have a happy ending. 'Once the dreaming changes, the morning mood changes,' she says. 'If people stop having unpleasant, guilt-ridden, anxious dreams, they wake in the morning more refreshed and better able to face the world.'

If you still feel grouchy and tired when you wake, despite having wonderful healing dreams, there could be another answer. Many scientists believe the Spaniards, far from being lazy, have had the right idea all along with their afternoon siesta. The body's circadian rhythms show that we are ready for sleep around 3 or 4 pm and that many overtiredness problems could be solved by a half-hour nap in the afternoon. Researchers have discovered that careful use of naps can help long-distance truck drivers, over-worked junior hospital doctors and residents, and those on night shifts; an afternoon catnap significantly sharpens mental alertness and improves mood.

What happens when we sleep?

Remarkably little is known about the actual physiological effects of sleep, but the facts, as they emerge, are intriguing. In the first 3 hours of sleep. large amounts of growth hormone are released into the body. Although the reasons for this in humans are not quite clear, growth hormone in animals is known to give immune systems a boost. As deep sleep ensues, more immune activities get under way. Levels of other hormones rise rapidly, too, such as prolactin, which is believed to regulate glucose and fatty acids in the blood, reduce water loss in the kidneys and generally balance our bodies. Melatonin, understood to influence regeneration and regulate water, is also released. So, while we slumber, our bodies appear to be fine-tuning, balancing and protecting.

Deprive yourself of the correct amount of sleep and you could find yourself becoming more irritable and antisocial. Your memory will not be as good and your coordination may be impaired. Your sex life may even suffer – research has discovered that our sex hormones are suppressed when we deprive ourselves of sleep.

Beating insomnia

Insomnia, the inability to sleep or sleeping poorly, often starts in infancy. Sometimes there are simple causes, such as bad habits or the effects of moving house. Sometimes, however, there is the deeper fear of separation. Parents who suffered childhood separation themselves often associate sleep with loss. Losing consciousness becomes frightening for them and they pass their anxieties on to their child.

As we grow up, our sleeplessness generally falls into three categories: transient insomnia, brought on by a change in routine such as jet lag or switching shifts; short-term insomnia, caused by illness or emotional problems; and chronic insomnia, which has myriad causes ranging from depression or anxiety to abuse of drugs or alcohol.

A doctor's standard response to 'I can't sleep' has often been simply to give a prescription for sleeping pills, but medical research is now showing that, far from being valuable lifelines, these drugs can cause more problems than they solve. Benzodiazepine drugs (such as temazepam, nitrazepam and triazolam) are most commonly prescribed, but research has shown them to be highly addictive. Withdrawal after long-term use can cause severe side effects such as cramps, vertigo, palpitations, panic attacks and seizures – not to mention rebound insomnia. Fortunately, doctors now view sleeping pills with more caution and are starting to use them only as a short-term rescue package for crisis management.

Try homeopathy

The following remedies are readily available from pharmacists or health stores. Take them in the 30x potency. Choose the remedy that most closely fits your symptoms. Of course, if you can, consult a professional homeopath.
- **ACONITE** for acute insomnia, caused by shock, fright, bad news or grief. You may be woken by nightmares and have fear, anxiety and restlessness. You feel better for fresh air, in a cool room, and feel worse at night, in a warm, stuffy room, with heavy or stifling bedclothes.
- **ARENSICUM ALBUM** for waking between 1 am and 3 am because of anxiety or an overactive mind. You are sleepy during the day, but anxious at night. You are restless in bed, with anxious dreams and nightmares. You feel better for warmth, warm drinks and sleeping propped up in bed, and worse when alone, cold or drinking alcohol.
- **CHAMOMILLA** for irritable babies who refuse to be calmed and sleeplessness caused by teething, anger or colic. They moan while asleep and their eyes are half open. They

feel better when carried or travelling in car, worse after 9 pm, after burping, in cold, windy weather and when too hot.

- **IGNATIA** for sleeplessness caused by shock, emotional stress or grief. You have mood swings, no thirst and your limbs jerk when falling asleep. You feel better for being distracted, worse for coffee and alcohol, cold and fresh air. You crave sweet things, but they make you feel worse.
- **LACHESIS** for menopausal sleep problems. You may feel suffocated or hold your breath as you go to sleep. You awaken suddenly and it may feel as if the bed is swaying. Night sweats and anxiety are common, and you may awaken feeling unwell. You feel better for fresh air, but worse for tight clothes and warm, stuffy rooms.
- **NUX VOMICA** for waking around 3 or 4 am feeling bright and cheerful, and not sleeping again until just before usual getting-up time. Your sleeplessness is due to irritability, overwork or working late. You are drowsy in the evening and after food, suffer nightmares, and feel better for warmth, in the evening and when left alone. You feel worse for alcohol, overeating (especially spicy foods), noise and lack of sleep.
- **PULSATILLA** for early waking with an overactive mind and/or recurrent thoughts. You have anxious or vivid dreams and night sweats, and throw off bedclothes feeling too hot, but then pull them back because you feel cold. You feel better for cool drinks and affection, but worse in a stuffy room.
- **SEPIA** for difficulty falling asleep. You wake up early feeling unrefreshed. You are exhausted and depressed by mental stress and overwork, and feel irritable and sleepy during the day. You suffer headaches, nausea and dizziness due to tiredness and night sweats. You feel better for naps, exercise and fresh air, but worse in thunderstorms or heavy weather.
- **SULPHUR** for awakening at the slightest noise and finding it difficult to get back to sleep. You feel hot and thrust limbs out from under the covers. You have vivid nightmares, disturbed and unrefreshing sleep, wake in the early hours and then sleep late. You are kept awake by a continuous flow of ideas. You feel better for lying on the right side, but worse for stuffy rooms and a hot bed.

Other alternative approaches

- Try yoga, meditation and breathing techniques – these can all help if stress is a factor.
- Relaxation or visualization tapes can often help you relax and sleep (try the exercise in the box at right).
- Acupuncture can alleviate insomnia and has been known to cure unpleasant dreams and nightmares.
- Hypnotherapy can help you to break bad habits.
- From the nineteenth century until the twentieth, in mental asylums, anyone who was particularly agitated would be put in a neutral bath. Have your bath at just above body temperature and, if you add Epsom salts, you can create your own home flotation tank. It has a very calming, relaxing effect, but you do need to spend a good half-hour there.
- White chestnut, a Bach flower remedy, can be very helpful if you can't switch off mentally. This remedy is specifically for thoughts that go round and round, and can have quite miraculous results. Put a couple of drops in water and sip.
- Herbs can help. Basil tones and calms the nervous system – it acts as a natural tranquillizer. Try pesto soup for supper. Valerian has been used to wean people off Valium and other tranquillizers. Take 1–2 g of the dried root as a tea 45 minutes before bedtime. Passiflora is also a soporific; try 1–2 g of the dried herb as a tea, as for valerian.
- Aromatherapy is very soothing. Use either a few drops of oil in the bath or on a tissue next to your pillow: use lavender, camomile and neroli to relieve anxiety and to calm, soothe and balance the mind and emotions. Use bergamot for insomnia linked to depression. Benzoin is useful when worries are causing sleeplessness. Clary sage

is for deep relaxation (but not to be used with alcohol). Marjoram, sandalwood, juniper and ylang ylang are all warming and comforting.
- A massage (ideally before bedtime or late afternoon) will often work wonders if you are suffering insomnia. Choose from the oils listed above as needed.

Winding down

This is a progressive relaxation technique.
- Lie or sit with your eyes closed in a dark room. Beginning at your toes, tense your muscles, hold for a count of three, and then relax them.
- Tense and release all the major muscle groups in the body, working from your toes and fingertips up to your neck and facial muscles.
- Breathe deeply as you do this exercise. Take a deep breath in through the nose, hold for a count of five, and then exhale slowly through the mouth while repeating the word 'calm' in your mind.

Solving insomnia – without sleeping pills

FIRST PRINCIPLES
- Look for any underlying psychological causes behind your insomnia and, if necessary, seek appropriate help (such as counselling, stress management etc.).
- Keep your room cool and airy.
- Avoid caffeine, alcohol and heavy meals late in the evening.
- Make sure your bed is comfortable and right for you.
- Ensure you get enough aerobic exercise, but don't exercise too close to bedtime.
- Have a warm bath and a milky drink before you go to bed.
- Avoid refined carbohydrates, sugar, alcohol, tea and coffee, carbonated drinks and excess bran.
- Avoid going to bed hungry – low levels of blood sugar in the brain can cause insomnia.
- Be careful of low-calorie diets – they affect sleep hormone levels and interfere with sleep.

Make your bedroom a sanctuary

Your bedroom should be a sanctuary from the world – a safe, secure place in which you leave the cares of the day behind. However, it seems that retreating to bed could actually be contributing to our stress and malaise. Any number of health problems can be caused by unseen dangers in bedrooms, ranging from allergies to headaches, from memory loss to depression. Here's how to turn your bedroom into a safe, soothing sanctuary.
- First of all, clear out the clutter (see page 92). Your bedroom should be calming to the mind, which is not possible if you have piles of work and mess around you.
- Try to avoid working in your bedroom. If this is impossible, place your desk or work-space behind a screen so that you cannot be reminded of work while you are in bed.
- If possible, keep bookshelves out of the bedroom – they distract the mind. Keep ornaments restrained as well; lots of knicknacks are distracting (and also attract dust).

Safety-proof your bed

It's frightening to think we may be snuggling down in the equivalent of a chemical factory. If your bed is made from chipboard or particleboard (pressed-wood shavings held together with resin), however, it may well be emitting dangerous formaldehyde gases into the air. Formaldehyde has been estimated to cause sensitivity in around a fifth of the population: symptoms include insomnia, tiredness, coughing, skin rashes, headaches and throat and eye irritation. It is also a suspected carcinogen (causing cancer). It's not just the beds either: many sheets are coated with a formaldehyde finish to help prevent wrinkling.

In addition, your mattress and pillows could be stuffed with polyurethane foam, which not only makes a pleasant home for allergy-causing dust mites, but has also been linked with respiratory troubles and skin and eye irritations. So what do you do?

- Choose iron or untreated solid-wood bedframes. Antique (or more than 10 years old) bedframes are an alternative, as most formaldehyde gas will have gone after 10 years.
- Choose sheets made from unbleached, percale or 'green' cotton for summer. Cotton flannel sheets are ideal for winter. If you can afford it, buy natural linen sheets.
- Think about switching to a pure cotton mattress – without flame-resistant finishes. Futon mattresses are also safe. Choose cotton-filled pillows.
- If you're sensitive to dust mites, buy special mattress and pillow covers to alleviate this problem.

Make your bedroom a pleasure zone

Remember that your bedroom should be a place of rest and relaxation. Keep that thought in mind as you decide what to include and what to exclude. As far as possible, keep your bedroom dedicated to sleeping – and, of course, romance.

- Make your bedroom as comfortable as possible. Heap the bed with sumptuous cushions and pillows (stuff them with herbs such as lavender and geranium for a good night's sleep).
- Choose soft, gentle lighting. Avoid harsh overhead lights and pick soft bedside lamps or uplighters instead. Candles work wonderfully in bedrooms; choose ones made with pure aromatherapy oils (rather than synthetic fragrances) for soporific scents. But do put them out before you sleep.
- Fresh flowers make your bedroom special. Choose scented flowers such as old-fashioned roses, lilies and freesias. Plant window boxes with night-scented stocks, lavender and camomile for sweet dreams throughout the summer.
- Buy an aromatherapy burner and scent your bedroom with your favourite scents – try ylang ylang, sandalwood, geranium or lavender for starters. Put a few drops of lavender oil on a tissue and tuck it by your pillow.

13

The Therapies

The Skeletal Structure

Osteopathy

Osteopathy is a system of massage and manipulation which aims to bring the structure of the body back into balance. Although considered a 'spine' therapy, it can achieve excellent results with a wide variety of conditions.

While many people think of osteopaths as simple bone-crunchers, that's a long way from the full story. Osteopathy was developed in the American Midwest in the nineteenth century, by a medical doctor and Methodist minister, Dr Andrew Taylor Still. He believed that by adjusting the structure, the framework of the body, its internal systems would be relieved and the body could then function properly and restore itself to health.

The philosophy underpinning osteopathy is that, if the anatomy and physiology are working well, the person is well. Sadly, we have a design problem working against us. In terms of human evolution, we have only recently made the transition onto two feet. Standing upright causes stresses and strains that our bodies have not yet adapted to: the discs between vertebrae have become weight-carrying and the continual strain can cause back pain and related problems.

The spine protects the major part of the nervous system, which, in turn, controls movement and registers sensations throughout the whole body. If the spine is badly aligned, symptoms might appear in any number of far-flung corners of the body. However, osteopaths don't focus just on the spine – muscular tension also needs to be relieved, as tension here can slow down the circulatory and lymphatic systems, inhibit heart function and worsen respiratory conditions.

Modern osteopathy uses a wide variety of techniques: manipulation and stretching, massage and gentle touch. In addition to these, your osteopath will often advise you on posture, diet and exercise.

What can osteopathy help?

- Osteopathy has good results with muscular and joint pain; frozen shoulders and all musculoskeletal problems.
- It is excellent for sports injuries and repetitive strain injury (RSI).
- Arthritic and rheumatic conditions respond well.
- Headaches and migraine can be helped.
- Chronic conditions such as asthma and bronchitis can respond well to osteopathy.
- Developmental problems can often be helped. So, too, can postural problems.
- It can be very valuable for the elderly.

- It can prove very useful both during and after pregnancy by helping a woman's body adapt to the considerable strains placed on it by pregnancy and birth.
- Some quite surprising ailments can be improved including digestive problems such as irritable bowel syndrome (IBS) and colitis, and menstrual problems such as premenstrual syndrome (PMS) and painful periods.

What can I expect from a session?

WHERE WILL I HAVE THE TREATMENT?
You will sit down to discuss your case with the osteopath, and then be asked to stand and walk around the room. The majority of the treatment will be conducted on the osteopath's couch, either sitting or lying.

WILL I BE CLOTHED?
Most osteopaths will ask you to strip down to underwear: You may be given a gown to wear.

WHAT HAPPENS?
You will be asked for a case history (precise details of your past and present health; any accidents, operations, and medication or remedies currently being taken; your life at home and work; your present problem and how it started, and what makes it feel better or worse). You will then usually be asked to demonstrate your mobility and posture – standing, sitting, walking up and down the room, leaning in all directions. Next, the osteopath will ask you either to sit or to lie down on the couch while he or she works on you.

Although massage may form part of the treatment, osteopathy is definitely not a pampering remedy and everything is performed swiftly and functionally. Often massage, deep stretching and pressure-point work (pressing deeply into the muscles and connective tissue) is enough to solve the problem.

You may also have to have your spine manipulated, a treatment in which the vertebrae are swiftly cracked to allow them to return to their correct alignment.

WILL IT HURT?
It depends very much on the osteopath! Some are very gentle and only use manipulation as a last resort; others really do crack and crunch your vertebrae, which can be a rather uncomfortable and unpleasant process. However, the sense of relief you will feel when a joint is returned to its correct alignment can be immense and it is well worth any slight discomfort.

WILL ANYTHING STRANGE HAPPEN?
You may well experience a feeling of flushing as the blood rushes into an area that has been constricted. Occasionally (although less so than in other bodywork therapies), you may also find that old memories resurface.

WILL I BE GIVEN ANYTHING TO TAKE?
No, medication is not part of the osteopathic treatment.

IS THERE ANY HOMEWORK?
Some osteopaths will give you exercises to perform at home to improve your posture or to help your problem. They may also advise you on diet.

HOME BACK CLASS
Osteopathy is a precise science and you should not attempt it at home. You can, however, use this simple back-stretching routine to help keep your spine supple. If you suffer from back or neck problems, check with your doctor before stretching.

You should feel a gentle stretch while doing these exercises, but not pain. Stop immediately if you feel any pain at all. Don't continue with the exercises; instead, consult a qualified osteopath, as you may have a back problem.

1 Lie on your back on the floor. Bring your knees up to your chest and clasp them with your hands. Then, keeping your whole body as relaxed as possible, pull your knees in towards your chest slowly. Hold for about 10 seconds, then release.

2 Position yourself on all fours with your hands directly under your shoulders and your knees directly under your hips. Your back should be straight. Now gently arch your back, as if you were a cat. Let your head drop and feel your pelvis tuck in. Hold for about 20 seconds and release. Repeat this process several times.

3 Sit on the edge of an upright chair with your feet placed firmly on the floor, quite widely apart. Slowly begin to bend forwards, until your hands drop to the floor and your head is positioned between your knees. Make sure your movements are very slow and smooth – you should feel a gentle stretch (if you do feel any pain, stop). Hold for about 10 seconds. This is an ideal exercise to practise throughout the day, especially if you have a sedentary job.

Cranial osteopathy & cranio-sacral therapy

The key to health and happiness may actually lie hidden in your head – not in your mind, but in the tiny joints that make up your skull. Cranial osteopaths and cranio-sacral therapists use the gentlest of touches to achieve remarkable results on these minute joints, called sutures.

There are two schools of cranial work: one practised by some osteopaths as part of their wider repertoire and the other a sideshoot known as cranio-sacral therapy, which is either performed as a therapy on its own or incorporated into other forms of bodywork such as shiatsu, massage and reflexology.

Both forms originate from the same source – the work of William Garner Sutherland. Sutherland trained as an osteopath in the early part of the twentieth century when osteopathy taught that the bones of the skull were firmly fixed together and immovable. Sutherland found, however, that the cranium was actually a moving structure. Its movements were certainly minute, but, like any other joint, the sutures of the skull ran the risk of becoming traumatized, restricted or stiff. Equally, also like any other joint, they could be manipulated back into balance.

Sutherland also discovered that there are certain rhythms in the cranium – a pulse that echoes the fluctuation of the cerebrospinal fluid (the watery liquid that bathes the tissues of the brain and spinal cord). When there is a problem in the body, or illness, this pulse stops beating at its optimum level of 10-14 beats a minute. Very gentle manipulation of the head and lower spine (the sacrum) can, however, correct the pulse and cure the problem.

Cranio-sacral therapy developed out of cranial osteopathy and is now a discipline in its own right. Unlike cranial osteopathy, its practitioners do not require any training in osteopathy or chiropractic. It was founded by Dr John Upledger, an American osteopath and physician who found that a large amount of cranial work could be taught easily and effectively to people with no background in osteopathy.

What can cranial osteopathy and cranio-sacral therapy help?

- A wide variety of conditions respond well to these therapies.
- They are superlative for babies, as they are so gentle and are particularly recommended if the birth was traumatic in any way (i.e. very swift, very protracted, with forceps or venteuse, or C-section).
- They can help a variety of problems from colic to feeding difficulties, poor sleeping to constant crying.

- They are also very useful for mothers after childbirth.
- Children respond particularly well – learning difficulties. poor coordination and hyper-activity can often be helped.
- Migraine, chronic headaches and sinus problems respond well. There has been success with cases of osteoporosis and tinnitus.
- Some digestive and gynaecological conditions respond well.
- Intriguingly, there has been considerable success in treating phobias with cranial osteopathy and cranio-sacral therapy.

What can I expect from a session?

WHERE WILL I HAVE THE TREATMENT?
You will be lying on the therapist's couch.

WILL I BE CLOTHED?
Cranio-sacral therapists will ask you to remain fully clothed. Cranial osteopaths may well want you to strip to underwear, so as to be able to observe the entire spine.

WHAT HAPPENS?
Sessions start with a full case history, with particular emphasis on any injuries or illnesses. A cranial osteopath will ask you to strip down to your underwear and then observe your posture before asking you to lie on the couch. The touch is very gentle and the manip-ulations minimal – a slight twist here, a gentle pull there. Most of the work is performed on the sutures of the skull while the osteopath cradles the head. The base of the spine (the sacrum) Is also held. The therapist's touch is so minimal that it is often hard to detect that anything is being done at all.

Cranio-sacral therapists use the same techniques, but usually keep you fully clothed. They often combine the treatment with guided visualization, colour therapy or on occa-sion, holistic foot massage. Sessions are much longer than those with cranial osteopaths and generally. more emotional and psychological (sometimes even mystical) In approach.

WILL IT HURT?
No, it doesn't hurt at all. In fact, you will feel only the tiniest, most gentle of touches. It is incredibly relaxing and soothing.

WILL ANYTHING STRANGE HAPPEN?
Some people find that images or colours 'pop' Into their heads while on the couch. It's not uncommon to remember past events or relive old and sometimes painful emotions.

WILL I BE GIVEN ANYTHING TO TAKE?
No, medication is not part of the treatment, although some cranio-sacral therapists may include flower remedies in their practice if they feel these will be beneficial.

IS THERE ANY HOMEWORK?
It may be that the therapist will teach you some techniques to practise at home.

Chiropractic

Chiropractors like to say that they practise bloodless surgery. Their aim is to maintain the spine and the nervous system (and hence the whole body) in good health and harmony, without recourse to surgery or drugs. Sometimes the results can seem like miracles – the chiropractor cracks a joint in the spine and a pain somewhere quite different simply vanishes. Although the name *chiropractic* sounds exotic, it simply means 'done by hand'.

The chiropractor is looking for a balanced spine that moves and functions harmoniously. If any of the individual joints move less or more than they should, or move in an abnormal way, the spine as a whole will fall out of its equilibrium and not work correctly.

Adjustments and manipulations help the mechanical function of the spine, which in turn helps muscles, nerves, joints and ligaments to work better. Chiropractors don't 'put bones back', as many people think; a bone only 'comes out' if it is dislocated. They prefer the word *subluxation*, meaning that a bone is out of alignment relative to the one below.

The first treatment using chiropractic in its present form took place in 1895 and was carried out by Daniel David (D. D.) Palmer, a Canadian schoolmaster-turned-store-keeper-turned-healer. Like many healers, he was driven to discover the true cause of sickness, as he believed that there is a fundamental reason why we become ill.

The start of chiropractic was quite dramatic. Palmer found that a man who had been deaf for 17 years also had a displaced vertebra. He put the vertebra back into position and the man's hearing returned instantly. Another case followed shortly: this time, once the displaced vertebra was replaced, Palmer found he had miraculously cured heart trouble. Palmer was fascinated. He began to theorize that all disease could be caused by an imbalance of tension in the nerves running through the spine.

Now, alongside osteopathy, chiropractic is probably the form of natural medicine most accepted by the orthodox medical world. Medical doctors quite happily refer patients to both osteopaths and chiropractors, recognizing that they have methods of treating the root causes of pain that doctors can only numb with drugs.

What can chiropractic help?

- Chiropractic is especially successful in treating mechanical problems of the spine, which can cause lumbago, sciatica, headaches etc.
- It is helpful in some cases of arthritis and rheumatism.
- Chiropractic promotes ease of movement in the chest and so can help asthma.
- It can be helpful In cases of Parkinson's disease, multiple sclerosis and some cancers.
- It can ease back problems and aches and pains in pregnancy.

What can I expect from a session?

WHERE WILL I HAVE THE TREATMENT?
You will start off the consultation sitting, while you talk to the chiropractor You will then be asked to stand for observation. The actual chiropractic work is carried out with you lying or sitting on the practitioner's couch.

WILL I BE CLOTHED?
You will usually be asked to strip down to underwear. You may be given an open-backed gown to wear throughout the treatment.

WHAT HAPPENS?
A full case history will be taken – you will be asked about your medical history, any past illnesses and in particular any injuries to joints or bones. You will also be quizzed on your present problem – your symptoms, when it's better and when it's worse, how long you've had it. You will then be asked to stand and sit, so your spine can be examined, after- which you will usually lie on the couch. Here, the chiropractor will test the mobility of your legs and will feel your spine to see if any joints or vertebrae are impaired. X-rays may be taken and possibly blood or urine tests.

The major work consists of adjusting the joints, using pressure and manipulation. You will feel a sharp click or crunch as the problematic joint is thrust back into position, or you may have to twist or turn your body into the correct position.

Chiropractic is a very pragmatic, down-to-earth therapy – ideal if you like a solid medical approach It is well recognized and respected by most doctors.

WILL IT HURT?
It depends very much on the chiropractor and on your own personality. Some people enjoy the cracks and crunches; others hate them. The treatment is not really painful more uncomfortable and a bit of a shock to the system!

WILL ANYTHING STRANGE HAPPEN?
You may experience a rush of blood as a joint is released. Very occasionally chiropractic can spark old memories. Some people find the results nigh-on miraculous – they walk out pain free.

WILL I BE GIVEN ANYTHING TO TAKE?
No, medication is not part of the treatment. Some chiropractors, however, do work alongside medical doctors, who may prescribe drugs.

IS THERE ANY HOMEWORK?
You may be given advice on preventative measures to stop your problem recurring. You may also be taught postural exercises and stretches to do to help your spine.

How to soothe a bad back

1   Exercise if you possibly can: this will help mobilize the back and strengthen the muscles that support it. However, if you do suffer severe pain, you will need to consult an experienced physiotherapist or exercise therapist. Don't overdo the exercise and, if you experience pain (as opposed to a gentle stretch), stop!
2   Try gentle systems such as Pilates and yoga. There is a branch of yoga known as yoga therapy which can help bad backs specifically. Always see a wellqualified teacher, rather than trying to learn it yourself from books or videos.
3   Make sure your posture is good. Invest in a special 'back' chair from a specialist store if you have to sit down all day for work. A good example is the kind of chair that entails a kneeling position, so encouraging the healthy spinal curve, rather than a slump.
4   Check your mattress. Many people suffer from bad backs because they are sleeping on the wrong type of bed. Your mattress should be firm enough to support you, without being too hard (many orthopaedic beds are too hard for comfort). Also ensure you change your mattress every four or five years.

McTimoney chiropractic

Although many chiropractors work very gently, there really is only one sure-fire way to be certain that your chiropractic treatment will never hurt and that's to find a McTimoney chiropractor. The McTimoney method seems to offer all the benefits of traditional osteopathy and chiropractic with none of the trauma. This holistic form of manipulative treatment uses a gentle technique to achieve harmony in the body.

John McTimoney, the originator of the system, was impressed by standard chiropractic, but felt that the system could be better still. First, he was convinced that the whole person should be treated, not just the part causing the problems. Secondly, he didn't see why the treatment should be uncomfortable or stressful. By experimenting, he found he could get the same, if not better, results by using very gentle techniques. In 1972, he started teaching his form of chiropractic. Although John McTimoney died in 1980, his students took up the baton and, in 1982, opened their own school to teach his work.

Many of us walk around with curves in our spines (caused by bad posture, carrying heavy bags, etc.). They are slight, but sufficient to cause twinges and pain. The McTimoney chiropractor aims to release these old patterns of holding, to wipe out bad habits overlaid on our ideal structure, so that our bodies can return to their original healthy blueprint.

The main technique used is called the toggle recoil. Basically, this involves the practitioner using one hand as a nail and the other as a hammer. The hands are held over the precise spot that needs treating and the 'hammer' is brought down sharply on the 'nail' with a slight twist. This action is rather like spinning a top and flicking it at the same time to set it moving. The effect is to change the tension surrounding the joint that has been 'toggled'. In a split second, the joint is freed: the adjustment is so rapid that it outwits the surrounding muscle, which does not have time to clamp fast into a protective spasm. The muscles are then able to relax and take up a more normal tension.

Because most of our holding patterns have been in place for years, most people tend to see McTimoney practitioners for around six sessions, in order to coax the joints to settle back into their natural position completely.

What can McTimoney chiropractic help?

- Most of the conditions that standard chiropractic alleviates – particularly joint and back pain – can be treated.
- Headaches, period pains and digestive pains often clear up.
- McTimoney chiropractic is wonderful both during and after pregnancy, as its manipulations can be safely used throughout – unlike standard chiropractic and osteopathy.
- Sports injuries respond well.
- There are special techniques to treat repetitive strain injury (RSI), carpal tunnel syndrome and tennis elbow.
- Many McTimoney chiropractors also treat animals with great success (under the auspices of a veterinarian).

What can I expect from a session?

WHERE WILL I HAVE THE TREATMENT?
You will be both sitting and lying on the therapist's couch.

WILL I BE CLOTHED?
You will be asked to strip down to underwear for the treatment.

WHAT HAPPENS?
You will be asked for a full case history, including the contact telephone number of your medical doctor. Expect to be asked about your medical history and current problem, as well as stress levels, sleep patterns, working conditions etc.

You will be asked to sit on the edge of the couch while the practitioner scans your spine. You then lie down, as the neck and pelvis are worked first. Small manipulations are then made to the knees, ankles and toes. The arms and hands are next to be treated, followed by the collarbone, face and skull.

McTimoney treatment always ends with a swift rubbing down, to bring you back to earth, as it were. As you sit up, your spine will be appraised again and it is possible the practitioner may feel it is necessary to make a couple more adjustments.

WILL IT HURT?
No, not at all. McTimoney is incredibly gentle.

WILL ANYTHING STRANGE HAPPEN?
It's not likely. The light 'swatting' feels a little strange to begin with, but it's not unpleasant.

WILL I BE GIVEN ANYTHING TO TAKE?
No, there is no medication, although some practitioners will refer patients to nutritional therapists if they think diet is a factor

IS THERE ANY HOMEWORK?
You may be given postural exercises and stretches to do, and recommendations on how to keep your body properly aligned.

Other forms of gentle chiropractic

Network chiropractic is a synthesis of all the varying forms of manipulation therapy. It is very gentle: nothing is ever forced. However much the practitioner might see the need to 'reset' a vertebra, he or she will not touch it until the body is absolutely ready, so relaxed that the adjustment causes no trauma whatsoever. Network chiropractors always look at the whole body, the whole person, rather than at individual vertebrae or bad knees. They seek to bring the entire body back into balance.

A study carried out at the University of California observed people who had undergone long-term network chiropractic. The subjects talked not just of physical improvements and pain relief, but also of more intangible benefits: greater self-esteem, more enjoyment at work and better family relationships. They reported feeling more motivated and felt more positive about the future. While such results are hard to prove scientifically, they seemed significant to the researchers.

BEST (bio-energetic synchronization technique) is another form of chiropractic. The job of the BEST practitioner is to update the neurology of the body. This is achieved by your lying fully clothed on the couch as the practitioner presses certain points while you hold your breath. Holding your breath means the brain cannot concentrate on anything except the need for oxygen so, as the point is pressed, the 'memory' held there is released. As you breathe out the body updates its neurological information – the old trauma is left behind.

WHAT DOES YOUR PAIN MEAN?
BEST chiropractic teaches that where we hold our pain can indicate the emotional problems we have:

Lower back pain concerns trust, confidence and security, or worries over your job, money or household environment. It also often relates to your relationship with your mother.

Middle-dorsal pain has to do with emotional/love relationships or low self-esteem.

Tense shoulders reflect self-expression – how you express yourself or how you deal with what people say.

Sciatica tends to affect people who can't stick by their decisions.

A stiff neck means you find it hard to listen to others.

Zero balancing

Zero balancing is a therapy that aims not merely to soothe and relax your physical frame, but also to stretch and balance your energetic body. It's a hands-on treatment which works physically at the deepest level of the body – the bone structure – and then moves deeper still, influencing the body's innermost energy systems.

Many therapies rely simply on bodywork, others focus solely on the energy part of the equation, but zero balancing (ZB) is based on the idea that better, faster, deeper healing can take place when the two are treated in tandem. It was developed by Dr Fritz Smith, an American physician, acupuncturist and osteopath who investigated a wide range of bodywork therapies and ancient energy systems before concluding that, in order to bring people from sickness to health, from imbalance to balance, he needed to combine the two approaches. The result was zero balancing, which first came into being around 1973. Smith calls it a 'blending of Eastern and Western ideas in terms of body and structure. It brings energy concepts into touch, or body handling.'

In zero balancing, energy is seen with clear precision. Three distinct types of energy surrounding the body are recognized, and a further three circulating within the body. Apparently, almost anything, from physical accidents to emotional traumas, can affect our 'energy' body. A blow to the knee can cause physical damage, but, long after the bruising has gone, the energy could remain twisted or stuck. Equally, an emotional shock such as bereavement or a relationship breakdown can remain caught in the energy web, causing not just psychological stress, but possibly physical stress and strain as well.

Zero balancers are all professional, highly trained bodyworkers. Before being accepted for training, they must already hold recognized qualifications in other forms of healthcare such as osteopathy, acupuncture, physiotherapy, chiropractic or Rolfing.

In many ways, zero balancing is the ideal therapy for people who feel nervous or uncomfortable about having to reveal too much of themselves. You won't have to take your clothes off, nor will you be expected to divulge your innermost secrets in painful soul baring.

What can zero balancing help?

- Zero balancing is often successful in curing headaches, and neck and shoulder pain.
- It is superb for alleviating back problems.
- Many sportspeople and performers rate zero balancing very highly.
- Although practitioners are cautious and won't make wild claims, many physical ailments clear up as a result of treatment.
- It has wide-reaching emotional effects – people often find they have more clarity and are able to make better decisions.
- Zero balancing has been described as akin to deep meditation: it takes people very deep into themselves so that the minor chitchat of the mind is silenced.
- It has good results on old injuries and any emotional troubles that have come about through past traumas and accidents. Emotional wounds -- such as bereavement or great disappointments – can often be healed quite easily.

What can I expect from a session?

WHERE WILL I HAVE THE TREATMENT?
You will be lying on the zero balancer's couch.

WILL I BE CLOTHED?
Yes. You need to take off only shoes and jewellery.

WHAT HAPPENS?

The zero balancer may ask if there is anything in particular that needs attention, and if you are suffering from any pain or stress. You then simply take off your shoes and any jewellery, and lie on your back on a couch. The practitioner works from the lower back down the legs to the feet, then to the upper back and finally towards the feet again. The touch sometimes feels like acupressure, shiatsu or osteopathy: at others, it is akin to Rolfing or Hellerwork. But it is unique.

The aim of the zero balancer is to get in touch with your energy system so that you can both work together on the problem. This approach is often known as the donkey-donkey touch because It's like two donkeys walking up a hill. If the donkeys are on a steep slope, they will lean into each other to help them get up the hill. Similarly, the practice of zero balancing is seen very much as a collaboration between therapist and client, rather than a treatment that a person passively 'receives'.

WILL IT HURT?

This all depends on your pain threshold. The touch used for zero balancing is pretty deep, but it is generally not painful. Although you may feel a little stiff after a session, this sensation swiftly passes.

WILL ANYTHING STRANGE HAPPEN?

You may feel curious sensations in the body or remember old incidents. Some people ' see ' colours or experience a buzzing in their heads.

WILL I BE GIVEN ANYTHING TO TAKE?

No, medication is not part of the treatment.

IS THERE ANY HOMEWORK?

You may be given postural exercises to do at home.

Sensing energy

As part of its teaching, zero balancing holds that the consciousness, or energy, of the practitioner can have a distinct effect on the person being treated. This exercise demonstrates how important this energy link is.

You will need a partner with whom to experiment to carry out this exercise.

1 Ask your partner to sit down in a chair and make himself or herself comfortable. Ask him or her to spend a few moments just quietly becoming aware of breathing calmly.
2 Now stand behind and rest one hand on his or her shoulder.
3 Both of you should bring your attention to the hand resting on the shoulder. How does it feel? Be aware of the pressure, the temperature, the 'sense' of touch.
4 After a few minutes, keep your hand in exactly the same position, but take your awareness away from your hand (you might look around the room or focus your thoughts on something entirely different). Tell your partner when you do this.
5 Now switch places – you sit down and ask your partner to repeat the exercise in exactly the same way.
6 Tell each other what you experienced, comparing sensations and feelings. This exercise is incredibly simple to do, but most people who try it are astonished by the results. When the awareness is taken away, there is often a feeling that the pressure lightens, that a sense of coolness replaces warmth (or vice versa).

14 The Fascia

Rolfing & Hellerwork

A session with a Rolfer or Hellerworker will transform the way you stand and alter the way you move. It could change patterns you have held for years, even since childhood. After a course of treatment (Rolfing has a standard 10 sessions; Hellerwork, 11), people's bodies quite literally look different – more upright, more centred, more relaxed.

At first sight, these treatments appear to be little more than a form of deep massage. So how do their practitioners achieve such dramatic results? The answer lies in the fascia, the connective tissue that encases every muscle and forms our tendons and ligaments. It keeps our whole structure, muscle and bone, in place.

Yet the fascial system had been generally ignored until the late 1940s when American biochemist Dr Ida Rolf discovered that the fascia would adapt to support whatever patterns of movement and posture the body adopted. If you put more weight on one leg than the other, the fascia will bunch and shorten to compensate. If you hunch your shoulders, the fascia will knot to accommodate and hold your posture. If we put our bodies into imbalance, the fascia will change to hold us in that position.

If they can change once, however, the fascia can change again. By manipulating and stretching the fascia back into their original positions, Rolf found she could reprogramme neurological pathways and return her patients to alignment. The benefit did not stop there. Rolf also found that, when she changed the body on a physiological level, her patients shifted on mental and emotional levels as well.

The other major deep-tissue technique is Hellerwork. Its founder, Joseph Heller, initially trained with Ida Rolf, but wanted to concentrate more on movement and the emotional side of treatment. As most Hellerworkers and Rofers will admit, however, nowadays the differences between these two bodywork systems are minimal and you will get equally good results with either one.

What can Rolfing and Hellerwork help?

- Postural problems respond best to Rolfing and Hellerwork.
- Long-term aches and pains often disappear.
- Chronic headaches can respond well to these treatments.
- Neck and back pains are usually alleviated.
- Energy levels are generally improved.
- Rolfing and Hellerwork can help improve athletic performance and general case of movement.
- There are usually psychological benefits, such as increased confidence the ability to deal with stressful situations and more honest relationships.
- Many people use Rolfing and Hellerwork to help them achieve personal growth.

What can I expect from a session?

WHERE WILL I HAVE THE TREATMENT?
You will be lying on a couch. Hellerworkers will ask you to move around as well.

WILL I BE CLOTHED?
You will be asked to strip down to your underwear.

WHAT HAPPENS?
The bodyworker will first scrutinize your body and posture as you stand in your under-wear. You may be photographed or perhaps videoed so that you will be able to see the difference at the end of your sessions. Hellerworkers will also spend time teaching you how to sit, stand and walk in a more balanced way. Each Hellerwork session has a theme such as 'inspiration' and, while the therapist is working, he or she will ask you questions such as: 'What inspires you?'

Both therapies are performed on a couch and the touch is virtually identical. It's Insistent and sometimes it can make you feel quite tender, but not unbearably so. It can feel wonderfully releasing, as old strains and stresses are stretched and straightened.

In the course of your 10 or 11 sessions, each part of the body is worked systematically a different part is worked at each session. With Hellerwork, each session also deals with a different emotional problem.

WILL IT HURT?
Of all the natural therapies, these have the reputation for being the most painful. The touch is deep and can thus hurt, but nowadays most deep-tissue bodyworkers will try to work within your pain threshold.

WILL ANYTHING STRANGE HAPPEN?
It's not uncommon suddenly to recall old memories, or for past incidents to come into your mind, both during and in the days following your session. You may well find you experience a surge of energy after treatment.

Physically, people say that they notice a change in their posture and their skin tone. More subtly, there can be distinct changes in the way people present themselves, their vitality, their confidence and their overall energy levels. If you have a high level of toxicity, you may find yourself feeling worse to begin with, as the treatment can release toxins held in the muscles and joints.

WILL I BE GIVEN ANYTHING TO TAKE?
No, medication is not part of the treatment.

IS THERE ANY HOMEWORK?
You may be given some postural exercises to do at home.

Rebalance your body

Try these simple exercises that will help to free your body:
* We often develop tensions because we are stuck in bad patterns. Try to break out of your habitual patterns by doing everyday things in a different way: try carrying your bag on the opposite shoulder from usual; throw or kick a ball with the opposite foot than normal; take your first step up stairs with the 'other' foot; brush your hair with the opposite hand. Although trying this strategy will undoubtedly feel strange, it will help to balance your body.
* Practise squatting whenever you can. Squatting is truly wonderful for the lower back and also helps to cure the scourge of modern life – constipation. Start gently and use

a table or chair for support as you lower into a squat. Getting up from a squat may be even more difficult than getting down: push into the ground with your weight over your feet, so that you don't strain your back.

- Give yourself at least 10 minutes of 'real rest' a day. Lie on your back on a mat or thin cushions on the floor. Your knees should be bent and your arms folded across your chest. Gently become aware of your breathing – don't try to alter it, just become aware. Feel it quieter, then focus on the out breath. Lie there, aware of your breathing and body. Roll over slowly onto each side before rolling over onto your front, onto all fours and then slowly getting up.

Bowen technique

There's no need to wind your head around any complex philosophy with the Bowen technique; no call for mystic mumblings or deep emotional encounters; no need to devote time to a drawn-out course of treatment. Quick, cheap and effective, it manipulates the muscles and connective tissue, leaving you walking tall and feeling relaxed, free and supple.

Bowen hails from the clean-living, no-nonsense, bright and breezy reaches of Australia. Its originator, Tom Bowen, studied medicine before the Second World War. By the 1950s, he was practising as a therapist, having developed a system of very precise, highly specific moves mingled with a liberal smattering of home remedies and almost folkloric advice. He allowed Oswald Rentsch to study his technique; after Bowen's death in 1982, Rentsch began to train other therapists.

The Bowen technique can be used on anyone, from the newborn to the elderly and immobile. A session takes just 20 minutes and you don't even have to take off your clothes.

Like Rolfers and Hellerworkers, Bowen practitioners work on the fascia, the connective tissue that covers the muscles, but with a quite different technique. It involves taking the slack across the muscle and moving over it. The touch is firm, but not painful. Around eight or ten prescribed moves are given in the first session, on the back and around the neck. Other moves can be used in later sessions. It may be simple, but Bowen is claimed to be highly effective: practitioners promise that 80-90 per cent of people need only one or two sessions to sort out their problems.

What can the bowen technique help?

- It is very useful for sports injuries in particular.
- Sportspeople also say it improves their performance.
- Lower back injuries and pain respond well.
- Chronic tension headaches often disappear after treatment.
- Problems such as asthma and bedwetting can be treated.

What can I expect from a session?

WHERE WILL I HAVE THE TREATMENT?
You will be lying on the therapist's couch.

WILL I BE CLOTHED?
Yes, you will be fully clothed.

WHAT HAPPENS?
You tell the practitioner your problem and then are asked to lie face-down on the couch. The therapist will start by working on your neck and back; you will feel a subtle

resistance and then a sense of 'giving way', as each muscle is 'rolled over'. It's a deeply satisfying therapy – you really feel it has 'hit the spot' but it's also very gentle. You may feel marginally worse after a treatment, but therapists prefer that you feel some change, whether good or bad. Most people experience a distinct sense of relief either immediately or in the day or two after treatment.

WILL IT HURT?
No, it doesn't hurt at all.

WILL ANYTHING STRANGE HAPPEN?
No, Bowen doesn't usually have any strange effects.

WILL I BE GIVEN ANYTHING TO TAKE?
No, although you may be advised on home remedies.

IS THERE ANY HOMEWORK?
You may be given exercises to do or suggestions for home cures.

Do-it-yourself Bowen technique

The Bowen technique has a host of weird and wonderful home remedies. These include:

For bunions – soak your feet in warm water containing about 3 tablespoons of Epsom salts every night for 3 weeks. The salts apparently break down the calcification that causes bunions.

For swollen knees or other joints – put crushed washing soda in a handkerchief, wrap it in a cloth and fasten this to the joint with a stocking before going to bed. The washing soda should draw out the fluid and the swelling should go down.

For bruises – apple cider vinegar applied to bruises or sprained wrists should take away the pain and tenderness.

For bladder problems and dizziness – take two slices (no more than 50 g/2 oz) of raw beetroot daily, in juice form.

For bedwetting – often the problem is psychological, but children who bedwet should avoid dairy produce, apples and apple juice and go on an 80 per cent alkaline/20 per cent acid diet. Bowen believed that apple juice weakens the bladder.

For arthritis – Epsom salts in the bath water can help.

For rheumatism – regular doses of honey mixed with cider vinegar can ease symptoms.

15 Pressure Points

Acupressure & Shiatsu

Acupressure is generally known as acupuncture without the needles. So, it's perfect for anyone who wants the benefits of traditional Chinese medicine, but is wary of needles. The theory is that vital energy, qi, runs through the body via channels called meridians. If the energy becomes stuck or sluggish, or races too fast, ill health will ensue. The aim of acupressure and shiatsu (the Japanese version) is to restore equilibrium to the energy flow.

Acupressure is old – very old. A form of it has been practised for perhaps more than 5,000 years. It is thought to have originated in India, then spread to Central Asia, Egypt and China, but it was the Chinese who took the system and made acupressure their own. For thousands of years, it was part of the practice of the folk healers known as 'barefoot practitioners' who travelled from village to village offering basic medical knowledge and the power of acupressure. The practice of shiatsu began in Japan around the sixth century AD; although very similar to Chinese acupressure, it has its own special characteristics.

These pressure-point therapies all work by stimulating the acupoints (tsubos in shiatsu) and so inducing the correct flow of qi or ki through the body. Physiologically, therapists say that they are shifting and diffusing the lactic acid and carbon monoxide that tend to accumulate in muscle tissue. These, they say, can cause stiffness and sluggishness in the blood which, in turn, affect every system of the body. Most therapists prefer to talk purely in terms of energy – allow the qi to flow smoothly and all manner of ailments will clear up.

What can acupressure and shiatsu help?

- These therapies are superb for stressbustIng.
- Emotional and psychological problems respond well.
- Chronic conditions such as back pain, migraine, rheumatism and arthritis can be helped.
- Asthma, constipation. Insomnia and sciatica can benefit.
- Acupressure and shiatsu often have success with impotence.

What can I expect from a session?

WHERE WILL I HAVE THE TREATMENT?
Shiatsu is always performed on a mat on the floor Therapists who use acupressure as part of other treatments will use a couch.

WILL I BE CLOTHED?

Shiatsu is always performed with the patient fully clothed (wear comfortable, loose-fitting clothes, ideally cotton). Other treatments may require you to strip down to your underwear.

WHAT HAPPENS?

Sessions start with a detailed case history You will then be asked to lie on the couch or floor on your back. An acupressure practitioner may read your pulses. A shiatsu practitioner will perform hara diagnosis – gently pressing your abdominal area to detect which meridians (channels of energy) are blocked and which organs might be under stress. Both techniques enable the practitioner to decide how to treat you. Specific points and series of points will be pressed – sometimes gently, sometimes quite firmly. In shlatsu, there may also be some stretching, in which your body will be gently pulled into position by the practitioner. At the end of the session, your pulses may be taken or your hara palpated again and you will finally be left on your own for a few minutes to 'come to'.

WILL IT HURT?

Some points can be quite tender – these are known as ahsi or 'ouch' points because people often say 'ouch' when they are pressed. Generally, however, these therapies are not painful.

WILL ANYTHING STRANGE HAPPEN?

It's not uncommon to feel a tingling or flushing effect as energy is released. You may find yourself 'seeing' Images as if dreaming, or having flashbacks to events in the past.

WILL I BE GIVEN ANYTHING TO TAKE?

No, medication is not part of these therapies.

IS THERE ANY HOMEWORK?

It's quite likely you will be given suggestions of things to carry out at home such as changes to your diet, postural exercises, breathing techniques or accupressure or shiatsu points to press.

Do-it-yourself shiatsu

Self-administered shiatsu is known as *do-in* and can be wonderfully energizing. Use this simple version whenever you feel tired or lethargic – it should give your batteries a good boost.

1 Tap all over the top of your head with your fingers. If you allow your wrists to become loose, you will find you are able to tap quite firmly. Use whatever rhythm suits you best.

2 Now place your hands on your forehead, with your fingertips meeting in the centre above your nose. Your elbows will be sticking out. Bring your fingers outwards to the edge of your forehead in a firm stroking movement. Repeat several times.

3 Using your fingertips, make little circles around your temple. Squeeze all along your eyebrows.

4 Next press firmly all around your eye sockets, but don't pull the skin.

5 Briskly rub your cheeks, then rub the end of your nose.

6 Press the points on either side of your nostrils (just under the nostrils there will be points that feel slightly tender). Press around your cheekbones with your thumbs, starting from the nostrils and moving round to your ears.

7 Pinch all around your ears. Gently tug your lobes. Rub all over the ears.

8 Pinch all along your lower jawline, from below the ears to your chin.

Seiki soho

Seiki soho is a form of bodywork that almost defies the imagination. It treats stress and strain, and has the uncanny power to 'read' your body, unravelling aches, pains and emotional traumas you barely knew you had. Practitioners of seiki soho describe it as 'a new technique using massage as meditation to enhance youthfulness, beauty and spontaneity', and explain that it helps you get in touch with your body and mind, clearing out the dross and leaving you free to feel good – in every way. This sounds a bit vague and seiki practitioners are the first to admit that seiki soho is short on theory and dogma. In fact, it actively avoids stringent philosophies and prescribed techniques.

Seiki soho was originated by a Japanese shiatsu practitioner, Akinobu Kishi (known as Kishi). He felt that shiatsu was too controlling – it sought to change the person's body, whether it wanted to change or not. His solution was to learn, though precise observation, exactly what the client's body wanted him to do. This observation is a skilled art and appears highly mysterious to the outsider. Practitioners say they can actually 'see' the point where a body wants to be touched. The belief is that all the troubling feelings and irritations of life become lodged inside us – about everything from traffic jams to unpaid bills, from unemployment to difficult relationships. While we can analyse them mentally, unless we bodily process and eliminate those feelings, they won't go away and eventually turn into physical ailments. Seiki clears the blockages, breaking old patterns of holding in muscle, bone and fascia.

What can seiki soho help?

- Seiki doesn't seek to cure; it aims to do what the body wants, so there are no particular conditions it can help, but equally none it cannot treat.
- It is almost universally relaxing and destressing, and seems to promote a deep cleansing effect on both body and mind.
- Many people find that, after a session, they feel both calm and energized, relaxed yet alert. They sleep better and feel better able to cope with the demands of modern life.
- It is especially suited for pregnant women. It fosters an even deeper bond between mother and unborn baby.

What can I expect from a session?

WHERE WILL I HAVE THE TREATMENT?
You will be lying on a large mat on the floor.

WILL I BE CLOTHED?
Yes, you remain fully clothed.

WHAT HAPPENS?
A case history is not taken, as particular problems are not treated. You simply lie down on the mat. The practitioner pauses for a moment, looking for problems areas, and then plunges in, working swiftly and assuredly. Many of the moves feel similar to the deep stretching of shiatsu, but there is no rigid system or pattern to the touch. You should become very relaxed. After an hour, you are left alone for a few minutes to 'come to' gently and then asked to sit quietly for a while sipping a glass of water.

WILL IT HURT?
The touch is firm and often quite deep, but not usually painful.

WILL ANYTHING STRANGE HAPPEN?
As with all bodywork, you may 'see' images or past events.

WILL I BE GIVEN ANYTHING TO TAKE?
No, medication is not part of the therapy.

IS THERE ANY HOMEWORK?
No, homework isn't part of the treatment.

Jin shin jyutsu

Jin shin jyutsu is an ancient Japanese therapy which works by balancing and harmonizing the body's vital energy, qi, through a series of 'safety energy locks'. The locks, of which there are 26 on each side of the body, are unseen regulators of our body's energy – they act almost like gears in a car. When the body is under strain, the locks can become congested and sore. Jin shin jyutsu aims to clear the locks so the energy can flow freely and the body helped back to optimum health.

You do not need long training or any experience for success. Many methods are so easy and unobtrusive that you can use them in a crowded bus – lots of jin shin jyutsu movements involve holds on the fingers and thumbs of the hand. Each of our fingers and thumbs can regulate 14,400 functions in the body, as they are connected by unseen paths of subtle energy to the rest of the body. By holding your fingers, you can affect any number of organs and bodily systems.

What can jin shin jyutsu help?

- A wide range of physical and psychological problems – headaches, menstrual pain, back tension, anxiety, depression, insomnia and even tantrums in children – can be helped.
- Some people say jin shin jyutsu can increase fertility.
- Do-it-yourself jin shin jyutsu can alleviate jet lag and it can help in many first-aid situations.
- Common ailments such as constipation, cramps and even bunions respond well.
- Practitioners don't aim to 'cure' anything – they simply harmonize the body into healing.

What can I expect from a session?

WHERE WILL I HAVE THE TREATMENT?
You will be lying on a couch.

WILL I BE CLOTHED?
Yes, you will be fully clothed, except for your shoes and watch.

WHAT HAPPENS?
Your qi pulses are taken to detect which locks are out of balance. The practitioner then lays one hand on a certain point of the body and the other on another point. The effect is like that of jump leads on a car battery – the practitioner acts as a cable for the circuit to clear.

WILL IT HURT?
When out-of-balance points on your body are held, you may feel distinct tenderness.

WILL ANYTHING STRANGE HAPPEN?
Some people find they start twitching or jerking under treatment, or that they start to smile or laugh as the locks are released.

WILL I BE GIVEN ANYTHING TO TAKE?
No, medication is not part of the treatment.

IS THERE ANY HOMEWORK?
Practitioners often supply a self-help programme to practise each day. They encourage patients to back up jin shin jyutsu with good diet, regular exercise and lymphatic drainage,

Self-jin shin jyutsu

This basic exercise will help bring your internal organs into balance. It can also help prevent jet lag – practise it during the flight whenever you fly.
1 Hold the thumb of your left hand with the fingers of your right and wait until you feel a steady pulse. This is your qi pulse, not the blood pulse.
2 Once you feel the pulse, do the same thing, but this time holding on to the index finger of your left hand. Again, stop once you feel the pulse.
3 Keep going, working your way through all the fingers of your left hand. Then swap over and do the same thing with your right hand.
4 You'll find that, as you practise, you will get quicker and quicker. Ideally, do this exercise every day in order to gain the maximum benefit.

If you're tense or irritable, this simple exercise can be performed discreetly.
1 Take the middle joint of your left middle finger lightly between your right thumb and fingers. Hold gently for a few minutes.
2 Swap hands, holding the middle joint of your right middle finger between your left thumb and fingers.

Reflexology

Reflexology is much more than just a foot massage. This ancient technique can bring your whole body back into balance and, practised properly, can have deep, effective results on a large range of health problems.

The theory is that every part of your body is mapped out on the feet. It may sound a strange idea, but it's certainly not a new concept. More than 5,000 years ago, the Indians and Chinese were using a similar technique, and evidence suggests that the skill goes back still further to ancient Egypt and even beyond. Pictographs found in a tomb of an Egyptian physician dating back to 2500-2330 BC show a man being treated with a form of reflexology. It is also a strong tradition in many African tribes and Native American peoples.

However, it was left to Dr William Fitzgerald, an American ear, nose and throat specialist, to popularize a 'new' therapy, which he called zone therapy, in the Western world in 1902. Fitzgerald first realized the importance of pressure on parts of the body when watching how pain could be relieved during surgical operations through pressure being applied to certain areas of the body. His work was developed still more by a fellow American, Eunice Ingham, who concentrated almost entirely on the feet and turned zone therapy into what we recognize today as reflexology.

Reflexologists realized that different areas of the feet and toes corresponded to different body systems: for example, the big toe relates to the head and brain; the rest of the toes represent sinuses; the lungs spread across the ball of the foot; and the lower back is down near the heel. By massaging the relevant point on the foot, the reflexologist is loosening tension and relieving blockages in the flow of energy to the corresponding part of the system.

On a more general level, the massage works to stimulate blood circulation and the lymphatic system, increasing energy and helping with the process of elimination of toxins. A more recent form of reflexology is the Morrell system, which was developed by Patricia Morrell, a UK reflexologist. She discovered that it was not necessary to press hard on the points: in fact, she found that a very gentle touch could have as good, if not better, results.

What can reflexology help?

- Reflexology can be remarkably powerful – in the right hands, it can affect almost all conditions.
- It is particularly effective for digestive disorders and constipation.
- Menstrual and menopausal problems respond well.
- Stress and fatigue can be helped.
- Migraines and skin conditions seem to respond.

What can I expect from a session?

WHERE WILL I HAVE THE TREATMENT?
You will be lying on a couch or, more usually, in a special chair .

WILL I BE CLOTHED?
Yes, you will be asked to take off only your shoes and socks.

WHAT HAPPENS?
A full case history will be taken before treatment. You then take off your shoes and socks, and lie down on the couch or chair often covered with a blanket. You are asked to shut your eyes and relax. The practitioner will examine your feet, feeling for any tenderness and looking for visual signs such as bunions, areas of hard skin and callouses, all of which tell a story.

The practitioner's thumb is mostly used to apply pressure. Reflexology can be a very strong therapy; you should always make sure your therapist is properly qualified (unfortunately, as with aromatherapy many people practise without proper training). If you are pregnant, never trust your feet to anyone other than a very experienced practitioner and only in later pregnancy.

At the end of your session, you will be left for a few moments to 'come to' and will then probably be given a drink of water and told to take it easy for the next few hours.

WILL IT HURT?
It is not generally painful, although some practitioners can be overly forceful. If you have a congested area, it will feel sensitive.

WILL ANYTHING STRANGE HAPPEN?
Afterwards, you may want to urinate far more than usual, or you may erupt in spots or perspire more (all signs of elimination).

WILL I BE GIVEN ANYTHING TO TAKE?
No, medication is not part of the treatment.

IS THERE ANY HOMEWORK?
You may be given some simple techniques to carry out at home, but usually you should leave reflexology in the hands of experts.

Self-reflexology

I am very cautious about self-reflexology. However, treating someone to this routine at home is generally quite safe (although do not give to a pregnant woman) and very soothing. Try it before bedtime for a wonderful night's sleep.

1 Gently warm some (plain, not roasted) sesame oil in a bowl.
2 Massage the right foot first. Pour some oil into the palm of your hand and then gently massage it into the foot. Use large movements to spread the oil evenly and well.
3 Now cover the foot in more detail, making small circling movements with your thumb. Work over the sole (firmly, if the person is ticklish), the heels and up to the ankles.
4 Sandwich the foot between your two hands and then massage with each hand moving in the opposite direction to the other – like the pistons on a train.
5 Circle gently but firmly all over the top of the foot.
6 Now pay attention to the toes – gently pull each one and massage.
7 Next work the following reflex points: the head, the solar plexus, the diaphragm and the heart. These lie across the tips of the toes and in band across the widest part of the sole of the foot. Use your thumb to hook firmly into each point, using the rest of your fingers behind the foot to balance your hand. If any point is tender, work carefully and within the person's pain threshold.
8 To finish, gently massage the centre of the forehead with sesame oil.

Watsu

Watsu is a deep, powerful and fascinating form of bodywork. A long, intense, intimate session of massage and manipulation techniques, carried out while you float in (or even under the surface of) a warm pool, watsu promises to heal you in mind, body and spirit. Fans claim it has remarkable regenerative qualities; that it can release stress, muscle tension and pain like no other treatment. They also say that it can equally release emotional anguish, giving you back a sense of childhood innocence and joy.

Watsu was the brainchild of Harold Dull, an American poet who became fascinated with shiatsu, the Japanese acupressure massage and stretching therapy. Having studied in San Francisco and Japan in the 1970s, Dull wanted to combine the therapeutic effects of shiatsu with the healing properties of water. He soon realized that he could achieve wonderful effects by floating his client in water, working on his or her body while cradling the head above water.

Several of Dull's students added their own twist to his idea. Jahara technique is performed much more slowly than watsu, with the client held further away from the practitioner. Floats are also used, making the whole experience less intimate. WaterDance was developed in 1987; like watsu, it begins with the client held above the water to be cradled, stretched and relaxed, but you are then given nose clips and gradually and gently taken entirely under the water. WaterDance is quite incredible to watch – the client moves underwater more like a dolphin or a mermaid than a human, somersaulting, rolling and undulating in complete freedom.

What can watsu help?

• Watsu takes the weight off the vertebrae and relaxes the muscles, giving greater freedom and mobility in the body.
• Watsu decreases muscular tension, increases superficial circulation and lymphatic function, strengthens the immune system and can aid digestion and respiratory difficulties.

- It is excellent for the later stages of pregnancy because it's so relaxing and water is so supportive.
- Many people find watsu helps insomnia and anxiety, and that it can release deeply held stress and improve posture. Watsu has achieved great success with sufferers of abuse.
- In California, it has been used successfully to help people with addictions and, paradoxically, it can even help people overcome a fear of water.
- It has profound effects on an emotional level, particularly with people who find intimacy difficult.
- The therapy is wonderful for children who have physical or mental disabilities.

What can I expect from a session?

WHERE WILL I HAVE THE TREATMENT?
You will be treated in a heated pool.

WILL I BE CLOTHED?
You will usually wear a swimsuit, although some people prefer to be naked.

WHAT HAPPENS?
The practitioner will ask you a series of questions. You then get into the pool, where the practitioner takes your head in his or her hands and asks you to lie back, relax and float. Throughout a watsu session, you are encouraged to breathe deeply and evenly, using only your mouth, and to keep your eyes gently closed. The breathing can feel a little unnatural to begin with; some people also find it strange and perhaps a little embarrassing to be cradled in the water by a virtual stranger. This feeling generally passes, however, and many people lose all sense of time.

As the water is so supportive, your body can be stretched much further than would be possible on dry land. There is a wonderful sense of release which comes over you as you are stretched, rocked and manipulated.

WILL IT HURT?
Watsu can sometimes be quite painful as stubborn tension is unknotted and leaves your body.

WILL ANYTHING STRANGE HAPPEN?
Many people find that when they leave the pool they are far more flexible and can bend far further than normal. It's also quite common to feel emotionally moved and even quite tearful. Being held so closely, particularly by a stranger, is simply not part of our culture and can be quite confronting.

WILL I BE GIVEN ANYTHING TO TAKE?
No, medication is not part of the treatment.

IS THERE ANY HOMEWORK?
No, homework is not usual, although some practitioners may suggest you adapt your diet or offer breathing techniques or exercises for you to practise.

16 Massage

Aromatherapy

Aromatherapy is probably the best-known natural therapy on offer and virtually every beauty salon will offer a version of this sweet-smelling therapy. Yet, true aromatherapy is much more than a sybaritic beauty treat – it's a powerful and far-reaching therapeutic tool.

Essential oils have a long and respected history dating back at least as far as ancient Egypt. Pots of scented unguents were found in Tutankhamen's tomb. Modern aromatherapy was 'born' in France in the early part of the twentieth century when Rene Maurice Gattefoss, a chemist, burned himself and discovered, by accident, that pure lavender oil could prevent scarring and infection.

About 300-plus essential oils are in use today. They are extracted from a wide variety of trees, shrubs, herbs and flowers. The oils work directly on the chemistry of the body: an essential oil contains on average too chemical components and chemists now know that they have myriad functions (for example, antibacterial, antifungal, antiseptic, deodorizing, digestive, antidepressant etc.). They are able to be effective therapeutically because they enter and leave the body with great efficiency, leaving no toxins behind.

Although it is clear that essential oils work in a direct way on the body's physiology, they also have more subtle effects. Scent works powerfully on mood – olfactory nerves connect to the limbic system of the brain, which regulates our sexual urge and our emotional behaviour. It also affects memory – in France, there are psychoanalysts who use fragrance to bring out the hidden memories of their patients.

What can aromatherapy help?

- Results are often most swift with any illness with a strong stress component. Aromatherapy is deeply relaxing
- Skin conditions respond well.
- It can strengthen the immune system and is useful for muscular pains and rheumatism
- High and low blood pressure can often be regulated
- psychological problems can be eased; It has good results with depression, anxiety stress and insomnia.
- It can be very relaxing in the later stages of pregnancy, but pregnant women must only be treated by a very well qualified and experienced aromatherapist.

What can I expect from a session?

WHERE WILL I HAVE THE TREATMENT?
You will be lying on the therapist's couch.

WILL I BE CLOTHED?
You will usually be asked to strip down to underwear or just briefs, but will be well covered with towels.

WHAT HAPPENS?

The aromatherapist will take a full case history – some oils cannot be used on people with high or low blood pressure or epilepsy. Others should not be used on pregnant women or those who are breastfeeding. You will then be left to undress and lie on the couch. The aromatherapist will decide on a mix of oils and make up a massage blend Some aromatherapists will ask you to sniff a variety of oils, believing that the ones to which you are drawn are those that you most need.

The massage itself is usually very gentle – the aim is not so much to affect the musculature as to apply the oils over the largest area of skin for maximum penetration. Most people fund they become deeply relaxed and it's not uncommon to doze off while you are lying on the couch

WILL IT HURT?

No, aromatherapy massage is usually very gentle.

WILL ANYTHING STRANGE HAPPEN?

It's highly unlikely. You should just feel incredibly relaxed and may even drift off to sleep.

WILL I BE GIVEN ANYTHING TO TAKE?

No. Very few aromatherapists use essential oils internally, as they can be dangerous if taken in this way. If your aromatherapist suggests this, ask if they are medically qualified.

IS THERE ANY HOMEWORK

You may be given some of the oil blend so that you can use it on yourself at home. You may also be given suggestions of oils to use in massage or in the bath.

Essential oils for home use

Always treat essential oils with great respect; if you're not sure of their effects, don't use them. That being said, these oils should be part of every home medicine cabinet. Always dilute oils: for a massage or bath oil, put eight drops of your chosen oil or oils in 4 teaspoons (15–20 ml) of a base oil such as sweet almond or walnut oil.

Geranium is a good-mood oil. Geranium lifts the spirits and can also alleviate insomnia and stress. It also helps to balance hormones and is useful for premenstrual syndrome. It can stimulate the lymphatic system and helps rid the body of toxins. Use as a massage oil or in the bath, or burn the oil in a diffuser. Lavender is a natural antiseptic; it's also wonderful for soothing burns. It acts as an antidepressant if you're feeling low and can soothe stress and insomnia This is one of the few oils that can be used undiluted.

Lemon is bright, fresh and tangy, and can help to shift cellulite and keep wrinkles at bay (or so they say!). It's a powerful bactericide and can help to stop bleeding, so use a drop or two of essential lemon oil in warm water on cuts.

Peppermint is a wonderful digestive tonic; if you're suffering from a stomach upset, massage your stomach with a peppermint blend. it's also useful in cases of shock – put a few drops on a tissue and sniff. A peppermint-blend bath oil will stimulate the brain and help you think more clearly – it's very energizing. Rosemary is an excellent tonic for the heart, liver and gall bladder; It also helps to lower cholesterol levels. Use it to ease colds, catarrh and sinusitis. It can help to soothe rheumatism and arthritis, or overworked or strained muscles – rub the diluted oil into the affected area.

Tea tree is a powerful antiseptic, antiviral and antibacterial oil – use it in your bath and in massage blends if you feel a cold coming on. It's useful for catarrh and sinusitis (put a few drops in a bowl of boiling hot water and inhale the fumes, with a towel over your head and the bowl). If you have an operation coming up, use it in your bath in the weeks prior to surgery – it will encourage swift healing.

Ylang ylang is a powerful aphrodisiac, use this oil in blends for a sensual massage.

Ylang ylang is also a wonderful relaxant and antidepressant, and it helps reduce high blood pressure

Hawaiian massage

Hawaiian massage has been practised in the Polynesian islands for centuries and promises to touch the part most massages fail to reach – your very soul. Practitioners say it can release hidden memories and spark change in your body, mind and soul. This massage can alter the way you think, feel, move and breathe.

Hawaiian massage (also known as huna massage or lomi lomi) is recognized in the USA as a byword for total pampering. Hosts of people (including many Hollywood stars) flock to Hawaii to put themselves in the hands of the kahunas. These are the native priests, acknowledged not only as great spiritual leaders, but also as superlative healers. They are taught that, in order to achieve perfect health and true happiness, you need to align yourself with the universal life force, to become one with creation. The massage acts as a gentle nudge, a reminder of how it is possible to feel at one with our bodies and, by extension, at one with creation.

The massage is known in Hawaii as the 'loving hands massage' and one of its key concepts is that the practitioner, often known as a performer, has to remain totally focused on the clients, feeling deep, unconditional love and compassion for them, rather than treating them as 'objects' to be 'fixed'. The training of a kahuna is arduous, long and steeped in mystery- few outside Hawaii have completed it. Now the kahunas are allowing elements of their work to be taken beyond the islands, however, and teaching outer aspects, such as the massage, to enlightened Westerners. Although the massage is but the simplest manifestation of the Huna philosophy, its effects can be deceptively powerful.

What can hawaiian massage help?

- Hawaiian massage affects the lymphatic, immune, digestive, circulatory and respiratory systems. It helps a wide variety of ailments, from irritable bowel syndrome to headaches and colds.
- It works deeply on the muscles, tendons and ligaments of the body, relieving aches and pains, and neck and back tension.

What can I expect from a session?

WHERE WILL I HAVE THE TREATMENT?
You will be lying on a couch.

WILL I BE CLOTHED?
It depends on the therapist. Some ask you to strip entirely; others will ask you to keep on your briefs and will cover you with towels.

WHAT HAPPENS?
Practitioners or performers practise in slightly different ways. Some will have the room temperature very high so that you can lie naked on the couch (as you would in Hawaii) Others tailor their work to a more traditional Western massage style – you can wear briefs and the parts not being worked are discreetly covered.

Some practitioners like to use volcanic stones placed down the spine to start the massage. Others will ask people to gaze at themselves in a mirror before the massage, trying to feel unconditional Jove for themselves.

The massage, however, always follows the same principles. Using light scented oils, the practitioner starts by massaging the back, sweeping down from your head right through to your legs in long, fluid strokes. The movement is rhythmic and repetitive and, after a few minutes, it becomes hard to sense where one stroke ends and the next begins, Practitioners throw their whole bodies into the work, often using not just their hands, but also the whole length of their forearm. As they pull, twist and stretch you, it feels as if you are partners in some strange dance.

At times, it feels like shiatsu and acupressure; at others, there's the firm but gentle feel of therapeutic massage, but the whole is far more than the sum of its parts. Almost every area of the body is covered, from the tips of your toes to the top of your head.

WILL IT HURT?
It can be quite deep and some points can be tender, but usually it's quite bearable.

WILL ANYTHING STRANGE HAPPEN?
It's easy to drift into a sense of total timelessness. Many people find that they shift from feelings of discomfort and embarrassment to ones of acceptance and connectedness. Some people have flashbacks to early experiences and it's not uncommon to feel intense emotions – people frequently report finding themselves either crying or laughing.

WILL I BE GIVEN ANYTHING TO TAKE?
No, medication is not part of the treatment.

IS THERE ANY HOMEWORK?
You may be asked to assess your lifestyle, diet and exercise.

Thai massage

Traditional Thai massage stretches you to the limit. Often called 'lazy man's yoga' or passive yoga', it lets you reap the benefits of stringent yoga postures without doing all the hard work – the practitioner flexes you into positions you would never have dreamed of reaching on your own. During a one and-a-half-hour session, your body will be bent and pulled, stretched and soothed. You will walk out feeling taller and looser, more open and expansive – as if every part of your body had been unlocked, allowing you to move and even breathe more easily, more freely.

Although still relatively new to the West, Thai massage has a long and venerable history. In the training schools in Thailand, they say it was developed more than 2,500 years ago in India by Jivaka Kumar Ell physician to the Buddha. Arriving in Thailand in the third century BC, the massage has been handed down from teacher to pupil ever since.

Like many Eastern massage systems, the Thai method works not just on the physical body, on unleashing tension in muscles and soft tissue, but also on the body's energy lines, the meridians. As an acupuncturist works with needles, so the Thai masseur works with his or her hands, feet and elbows to release blockages in the energy flow and to allow vital life force, qi, to run smoothly around the body once more. The result, they say, is improved flexibility, better circulation of blood and lymph, and an exhilarating dose of vitality.

What can thai massage help?

- Many people report that it has helped them considerably with headaches and sinus conditions.
- Stress and exhaustion caused by overwork respond well.
- Thai massage alleviates anxiety and depression, Linda whole host of emotional problems.
- The massage loosens the body, ameliorating deep-seated aches and pains.
- It seems to help people become more open and better able to communicate

What can I expect from a session?

WHERE WILL I HAVE THE TREATMENT?
You will be lying on a mat on the floor.

WILL I BE CLOTHED?
You will be asked to take off your shoes, socks and any jewellery, but otherwise stay fully clothed (ideally, wearing loose-fitting, comfortable clothes).

WHAT HAPPENS?
You will be asked if you are pregnant, or have a severe back problem or high blood pressure: if so, the massage can be adapted to suit your condition. The treatment starts at your feet, with your toes being bent back repeatedly. After the feet have been thoroughly stretched, the practitioner moves up the legs, round the hips and on to the stomach, using a pushing motion with his or her fingers.

Next come spinal stretches. With your knees bent one way and the practitioner pushing your shoulder in the opposite direction, you may well find your vertebrae starting to crack and crunch. Because the practitioner's body weight is gently rocking you into exactly the right position, the stretch goes much further than you could ever achieve on your own.

No part of the body is ignored in Thai massage – it really is a top-to-toe affair. Your hands, arms and shoulders receive the stretching treatment, and tension in the face and head is soothed by gently but firmly pressing on the pressure points. You are then pulled into a sitting position and the serious stress points in the neck and shoulders are addressed.

Some practitioners end with a special technique known as 'massage without touching', in which they sit behind you and, breathing swiftly and deeply, move their hands up and down the spine, without actually touching the body. Mysteriously, you feel an incredible tingle running throughout the body, a little like being hosed down with a powerful shower of water.

WILL IT HURT?
Sometimes the practitioner hits sore or particularly tense spots, which can feel a little tender, but generally the experience proves a very relaxing one.

WILL ANYTHING STRANGE HAPPEN?
At times it feels as if you are being stretched and manipulated by two or three people, but it's just that the practitioner is using his or her feet or elbows, as well as hands, to lend extra stretching power to the treatment.

WILL I BE GIVEN ANYTHING TO TAKE?
No, medication is not part of the treatment.

IS THERE ANY HOMEWORK?
No, you will not have any homework.

Chavutti thirumal

Chavutti thirumal (often known as the Indian rope massage) is practised with the feet, rather than the hands. While the idea may sound strange and even unpleasant, the reality is quite different. This is one of the deepest and yet most subtle of massage therapies: it feels heavenly and bestows prodigious health benefits.

Chavutti thirumal originated in South India and was developed primarily to keep practitioners of both the local martial arts and dance supple and flexible. Dancers and fighters would be given a 10-day intensive course of the massage before performances to enable them to perform in peak condition. It generally prevented injuries and strains, but, if anything did go wrong, a further course would equally coax them back to health.

The massage affects people in different ways. Some find the effects are all physical, while others find it affects them psychologically as well. Some people bounce away feeling on top of the world; others feel calm and centred. Some people actually feel worse before they feel better. This, say practitioners, is because the therapy draws things out. It can help eliminate toxins, too, which means people can sometimes suffer sore throats or headaches. But these side effects are short-lived.

Chavutti reaches every external muscle and ligament in the body, while stimulating the circulation and the lymphatic system. Stimulating the lymphatic system inevitably helps push toxins to the lymph nodes to be eliminated. It is this elimination that leads people to say that chavutti thirumal can be a factor in successful weight loss and even rejuvenation. In addition, the deep, kneading action is said to promote the breakdown of cellulite.

Today, chavutti thirumal has a small but fervent band of Western devotees. Because the massage is long (at least one-and-a-half hours), it is incredibly satisfying. The feet are, surprisingly, not clumsy at all and can do all that hands can do – and more. As the practitioner is standing (balancing his or her weight on a rope slung across the room), he or she can use much greater pressure if need be and really attack deep-seated tension and stress. The massage is much loved by overworked businesspeople, sportspeople and performers.

What can chavutti thirumal help?

- It is very helpful for muscle spasm or back tension.
- It's ideal for sportspeople, dancers, martial-arts practitioners and performers who need to keep their bodies supple and in tiptop condition.
  Practitioners say that the massage can help improve body image and encourages you to foster a sense of acceptance of your body, however imperfect.
- It can help troublesome emotions to clear and can sometimes relieve psychological blocks.
- It stretches every external muscle and ligament in the body while stimulating the circulation and the lymphatic system, helping toxins to be transported to the lymph nodes for elimination. This has led many people to claim the massage has helped them lose weight and feel rejuvenated.
- The deep, kneading action is said to promote the breakdown of cellulite.
  It can help alleviate the ill effects of overexercising and strained and sprained muscles.
- It is deeply stress relieving and can help any condition that has a stress-related background.

What can I expect from a session?

WHERE WILL I HAVE THE TREATMENT?
You will be lying on a line of rush mats on the floor with a large towel down the middle. Strung across the room, at head height, will be a thick red rope.

WILL I BE CLOTHED?
Usually, you will be asked to strip entirely. Some practitioners will give you a loincloth to wear. This may feel strange at first, but, once the treatments starts, you will forget about anything so mundane! The room is kept very warm, so you will not get cold.

WHAT HAPPENS?
The practitioner asks a few questions about any health problems, then prepares himself or herself. Practitioners regard chavutti thirumal as a spiritual exercise, so spend a few moments in prayer and meditation before the session. Throughout the massage, they breathe deeply to keep their energy channels open.

Your body is liberally doused with warm sesame oil and then, using the rope for balance and to modulate his or her weight, the practitioner starts to massage. The feeling is wonderful – strong, deep, yet highly sensitive. The feet are used expertly to knead, probe, stretch and soothe every muscle and ligament in the body – from the shoulders down to the toes, before ending up with your face and head. By the time the massage is finished, you will feel totally refreshed and yet relaxed.

WILL IT HURT?
The massage is very strong and tense muscles can feel quite sore. On the whole, however, it is a delicious experience.

WILL ANYTHING STRANGE HAPPEN?
You may find the breathing of the practitioner (which is fairly loud) rather strange to initially. At the end of the session, the practitioner usually spends a few moments working with your energy, with his or her hands off the body, something which can feel slightly odd after such an intense body workout.

WILL I BE GIVEN ANYTHING TO TAKE?
No, medication is not part of the treatment.

IS THERE ANY HOMEWORK?
No, you won't be given any homework.

Indian head massage

Indian head massage has been practised in India for thousands of years. Children are massaged from birth by their mothers and learn early how to give massages to the rest of the family. By the time they reach adulthood, they know It as a well-established family ritual.

Women have head massages to keep their hair beautiful and glossy; the men have it to prevent them from going bald. Everyone enjoys it as a supreme stressbuster and particular techniques can help prevent headaches and treat insomnia. Above all, because this massage can easily be learnt and shared, it has the valuable capacity of being able to bring both partners and families closer together. As Indian head massage expert Narendra Mehta explains: Touching makes us feel nurtured, cared for and relaxed. If husbands and wives could massage each other, even just on the top of the head, it would bring them closer.'

Originally, head massage was part of the system of ayurveda and was practised therapeutically; however, over the years the techniques were watered down and altered. Before the advent of barbers' and hairdressers' shops, barbers used to visit the homes of Indian families. Among their techniques, they introduced head massage, which not only improved the quality of their clients' hair, but also made them deeply relaxed. Sometimes the barbers took advantage of this deeply relaxed state and some were even renowned as spies who extracted secrets from their clients when they were utterly at ease after the massage!

The tradition of head massage has continued up to this day in India. It's quite common to find masseurs offering head massages on the beach, on street corners and even in busy markets. Quite apart from its cosmetic benefits, head massage is uniquely powerful as a stressbuster. The head, neck and shoulders (which are also included in a massage) are classic places in which we hold stress and so massage can be an easy, swift and effective way of preventing tension from building up in your body.

NOTE: Almost anyone can benefit, from the very young to the elderly. The only people who are not advised to have Indian head massage are those with weeping eczema or head injuries, the psychotic or those with epilepsy.

What can Indian head massage help?

- The massage improves blood flow to the brain – many businesspeople swear that it helps their performance, making them more alert and better able to concentrate.
- It alleviates anxiety and improves mood.
- Tension headaches and eye strain respond well.
- Indian head massage can help insomnia.
- The oil and massage improve the texture of your hair, giving a wonderful shine.
- Regular massage is said to help stop hair falling out and prevent it turning grey!
- It deeply relaxes the face muscles, making you look healthier and happier.

What can I expect from a session?

WHERE WILL I HAVE THE TREATMENT?
You will be sitting in a comfortable chair.

WILL I BE CLOTHED?
Yes, although some people prefer to take off their top or shirt in case the oil stains clothing.

WHAT HAPPENS?
Treatment starts with a deep kneading and probing of the neck and shoulder muscles Sometimes the treatment seems almost akin to osteopathy. but there is no crunching or cracking.

The therapist then moves on to the head The scalp is squeezed, rubbed, tapped and prodded; your hair is tugged and then 'combed' with the therapist's fingernails. The jawline is worked and ears are pulled, tugged and pressed.

Finally, the therapist moves to the face, pressing acupressure points to relieve sinus pressure, stimulate blood circulation and increase alertness. The face is then gently stroked.

WILL IT HURT?
Some points may be tender or sore, but generally the treatment feels divine.

WILL ANYTHING STRANGE HAPPEN?
The touch is so gentle that it can seem almost too intimate for some people. Some find it releases feelings of past hurt and a grieving for lost childhood.

WILL I BE GIVEN ANYTHING TO TAKE?
No, medication is not part of the treatment.

IS THERE ANY HOMEWORK?
Not specifically, although you may be taught massage techniques to practise at home; many people in fact go on to learn how to practise on friends and family.

Getting a head start at home

Indian head massage is one of the simplest techniques of massage to learn. You can easily give a highly effective treatment. Use either sesame or coconut oil. It should be warm but not hot – stand it on or near a heater for around half an hour, or place it in a microwave for a minute.

NOTE: Do not perform head massages if your subject has a skin condition such as weeping eczema or psoriasis, or there are open cuts or sores on the head.
  1 Have your subject sit upright in a straight-backed chair. Gently lay your hands on the crown of his or her head; hold them there for about 30 seconds. Slowly begin to

massage the scalp with the pads of your fingertips. If using oil, apply it now. Don't drench the hair: use just enough to lubricate the scalp. This gives a connection between you and your subject, putting you both at ease.

2   Progress to a technique known as 'windscreen wiper'. Support the head with one hand. Using the palm of your other hand, employ a swift rubbing motion, as if you were buffing a window. Start behind the ear, going around it and then away Repeat on the other side of the head. This relaxes and warms the muscles.

3   Next support the head with one hand while the other gently strokes the top of the head. Use long, sweeping motions first, then 'comb' the hair, running your finger-nails through the hair in long strokes. Work all the way around the head, swapping hands where necessary. This stimulates blood flow through the scalp, giving a lovely tingly feeling to the head.

4   Take the weight of your partner's head on your arm. Starting at the top of the neck (where it joins the cranium), massage down either side of the spine, using small circling movements of the thumb and middle finger. Go carefully and be aware of how your subject reacts – don't press too deeply. This stroke soothes and calms the brain itself.

5   Massage the temples using gentle circular movements – use the tips of the index fingers. Then support the back of the head with your hands and employ a firmer but still soft pressure, massaging the temples with your thumbs.

6   Now concentrate on the neck and shoulders. Imagine you are ironing the shoulders, using the heel of your hand to roll forwards over the shoulder from the back to the front. Start from the outside edge of the shoulder and move in towards the collar-bone. If you are performing the massage on someone much taller than you, use your forearm to press across the shoulder, deploying your body weight for pres-sure. This is wonderful for releasing tension in the shoulders and neck.

7   Put both hands around the head to form a cap Squeeze, lift and let go several times You can use this movement alone to combat headaches.

8   Now stroke the face lightly with the whole of your hands (palm against the face), moving gently down from the forehead to the chin. Repeat as much as you like. Cover the eyes with your palms, then press very gently on the eyeballs. If performing the massage before bedtime, it is best place to end here as it will send your subject gently off to sleep. This step done on its own can help treat insomnia.

9   If your subject wants to feel energized, finish with a brisk rubbing motion back and forth across the scalp. Vary this with a fast scratching action, using your fingernails. Both can be firm and deep. Finish by pressing firmly but carefully on the crown, as at the beginning.

Manual lymphatic drainage

Manual lymphatic drainage (MLD) combines pure bliss with deep healing. It's a gentle massage technique that encourages the elimination of toxins and the stimulation of the lymphatic system. MLD is now being recognized as an essential part of treating oedema (swelling); it is highly effective at bringing down oedema after surgery and after radio-therapy and chemotherapy for cancer. However, it's not just a medical treatment: MLD is also one of the bestkept secrets on the beauty scene.

Dr Emil Vodder and his wife Estrid developed MLD in France in the 1930s. Vodder noticed how people suffering from chronic catarrhal and sinus infections tended to have swollen lymph glands and, going against medical practice at the time, started to work with the lymph nodes. The massage the Vodders developed has a circular, pumping effect which increases the efficiency of the body's lymphatic system (which acts as the body's garbage disposal system). By helping to clear the body of debris and old toxic waste, MLD makes your skin look brighter and healthier on the outside, while inside your immune system is given the chance to function at optimal levels, offering your body protection against colds, flu and other illnesses.

The medical establishment is beginning to take MILD very seriously. If a massage is given to burns victims soon after the accident, it can rapidly reduce the burn. Scar tissue can be encouraged to build up only where needed, preventing large, unsightly scars. The therapy is often used on cancer patients, post-operatively, to limit the oedema that can arise.

People also visit MLD therapists for cosmetic reasons – MLD draws the skin in and tightens it. While it won't actually make you thinner, it will certainly make your face *look* thinner by tightening up all the little saggy, baggy bits, all the unsightly puffiness. It's rather like a mini facelift without surgery.

What can manual lymphatic drainage help?

- It can stop a cold in its tracks in many cases, or certainly reduce the symptoms.
- Sinus problems respond very well.
- MLD can improve your immune system in general, making you less susceptible to infections.
- Oedema (swelling) comes down dramatically. MLD is very useful in treating lymphoedema, which often develops after mastectomy or surgical removal of the lymph nodes, or following radiotherapy treatment.
- This therapy has wonderful effects on scar tissue and burns. Stretch marks and acne scarring can be cleared or diminished with commitment
- Some people say it can reduce cellulite. MLD is also sought of as a quasi-heathy treatment to firm facial tissue.

What can I expect from a session?

WHERE WILL I HAVE THE TREATMENT?
You will be lying on the therapist's couch.

WILL I BE CLOTHED?
You will be asked to strip down to your underwear but will be covered by towels throughout the session.

WHAT HAPPENS?
A full case history will be taken and the therapist will check that you haven't had tuberculosis and don't have heart problems. You will be quizzed not just on your medical history but also on your lifestyle. Then you will be left alone to undress and get on the couch.

The MLD touch is unique – it is a very gentle touch, rather like having your skin stroked by a child's gentle fingers. It involves a light, repetitive movement that has an almost hypnotic effect. In fact it can switch the body's nervous system to its relaxed 'night-time' mode.

After the massage, you will be left on the couch to relax for 5 minutes or so, before being given a glass of water to drink.

WILL IT HURT?
Absolutely not. This is about the most gentle kind of massage you could ever experience.

WILL ANYTHING STRANGE HAPPEN?
After the treatment, you may find your glands feel slightly swollen or uncomfortable – a sign that toxins are moving to the lymph nodes. You may be surprised at how much brighter and lighter your skin looks and feels. Any sniffles or stuffiness may vanish.

WILL I BE GIVEN ANYTHING TO TAKE?
No, medication is not part of this treatment.

IS THERE ANY HOMEWORK?
You may well be given guidelines on healthy eating and exercise. For the best results, you should practise MLD on yourself regularly – the therapist will show you how to do it.

Ways to ease the load on your lymphatic system

You need to be shown MLD by a trained therapist, but there are lots of other things you can do to help your lymphatic system detoxify.

Walk and swim – exercise acts as a powerful pump for the lymphatic system, but high-powered aerobics may be counterproductive as it earn overuse the muscles, creating more waste products. Swimming and walking are both superb.

Bounce – perhaps the best way to get your lymph moving is by bouncing on a small trampoline (a rebounder). Just 5 minutes a day will make a significant difference.

Eat well – high-fat diets (particularly dairy procure and red meat) encourage a buildup of toxins. Make sure your diet is rich in green vegetables, fresh fruits and sprouted seeds.

Drink water – make sure you drink al least 2 litres (2 quarts) of fresh spring water every day. Warm water can be helpful, too (keep a flask near to hand).

Skin brush – skin brushing moves the lymph and softens impacted lymph mucus in the nodes. Use a natural-bristle brush and brush smoothly, always moving towards your heart.

Try yoga – yoga positions, combined with deep breathing, help the lymphatic system. Head stands and other inverted positions are particularly good. If you find it tough to stand on your head or shoulders, lie down with your legs up the wall.

Use rosemary – put a couple of drops of rosemary oil (in a base oil) in a warm bath and relax Gradually add cool water until the water is quite cold – this change of temperature helps to stimulate the lymphatic system.

Chua ka

Chua ka is a form of deep-tissue bodywork with effects similar to those of therapies such as Rolfing and Hellerwork – although it achieves its results without quite so much discomfort. Chua ka is rumoured to have originated from a ritual used by ancient Mongolian warriors before battle to cleanse their bodies physically and prepare their minds for the mental and spiritual ordeal ahead. It's a great story, but one which, sadly, can't be proven. What is certain, however, is that, in its current form, chua ka was developed by an American, Oscar Ichazo, in the 1960s, as a result of his research into physiology and psychology. What is also crystal-clear is that, whatever its origins, chua ka is a highly effective massage technique. Better still, you can learn how to perform chua ka on yourself so that you can reap the benefits at any time.

Chua ka is a deep, detoxifying therapy. Ichazo believes that we were born as smooth and supple human beings. With age and the stress of life, however, we lose this elasticity and start to build up deposits on both the physical and emotional level Physically, these are made up of metabolic waste products. Equally, if not more, toxic, however, are memories of pain – whether physical, emotional, mental or even spiritual. Say, for example, you fell off a bicycle as a child, you might simply suffer a physical bruise and forget about it. But if you were surrounded by a crowd of children laughing at you, you could develop a 'psychic bruise' and store the memory in the muscle and connective tissue. Hence it's not uncommon when receiving deep-tissue massage such as chua ka to find old memories resurfacing quite unexpectedly.

What can chua ka help?

- Chua ka can be highly effective in treating back pain.
- Stress-related problems such as insomnia respond well.
- It is useful for digestive problems.
- Some people swear that it has helped reduce cellulite.
- Some chua ka practitioners have been able to help people with ailments as varied as rheumatoid arthritis, foot injuries, acne and bowel problems.
- In New York, politicians and models often have chua ka on their faces before television slots or photographic shoots, as it reduces puffiness and gives a form of 'Instant facelift'.
- It also has a strong psychological effect, working to heal emotional wounds and helping people deal with fear.
- Many people use it as a self-help tool for greater self-awareness.

What can I expect from a session?

WHERE WILL I HAVE THE TREATMENT?
You will be lying on a couch.

WILL I BE CLOTHED?
You wear just briefs, but are well covered with towels.

WHAT HAPPENS?
On the first visit, time is spent taking a history of your health, diet and lifestyle. Treatment can then be tailored to suit your needs or medical condition. The technique is unusual: long, slow, fluid strokes that probe deeply into the body, stimulating the circulatory system and helping the body regain some of its original elasticity. Strong pressure movements with the thumbs are also used to work into the deep tissue, releasing physical tension and stored trauma. Chua ka has aptly been described as 'reflexology for the body' – it feels as though the therapist is hitting every acupressure point in turn. Typically you could expect the therapist to work on your back, shoulders, arms and legs, ending with some deep work on your neck and some powerful pressure on your scalp and face.

WILL IT HURT?
At times it can be almost painful, but the pain is forgotten as your body releases its tension. It's that weird kind of 'good hurt'. If you are very sensitive to strong pressure, however; this may not be the best form of bodywork for you.

WILL ANYTHING STRANGE HAPPEN?
You may relive old hurts or find buried memories surfacing.

WILL I BE GIVEN ANYTHING TO TAKE?
No, medication is not part of the treatment.

IS THERE ANY HOMEWORK?
You may be asked to adjust your lifestyle, diet and exercise habits.

Trager®

Trager® or Trager Psychophysical Integration (to give it its full name) is a gentle system of bodywork, the predominant goal of which is to make life easier, more comfortable and more pleasurable. It helps you build up deep stores of energy and vitality, and yet keeps you calm and centred. In a typical session, you receive several thousand light, rhythmical touches and get up off the couch feeling like a child who has been rocked in its mother's arms.

The history of this deeper-than-deep relaxation treatment started back in the 1930s. Milton Trager was a young boxer and acrobat in Miami, Florida, intent upon training his superathletic body. He was always pushing himself to the limits, aiming to jump the highest, the farthest, to be the best. One day, he suddenly had a completely new thought. 'How can I land softer?' he pondered. Then: 'How could I land the softest?' His whole philosophy changed overnight – from aiming for maximum effort, he sought instead to achieve maximum effortlessness, to become ever lighter, easier, softer and freer. Trager discovered he could introduce the same feeling of ease and comfort to others by means of gentle rocking and stretching, and this became his life's work.

Over the next 40 years, he perfected Trager. Keen to put his ideas on a firm scientific footing, he trained and qualified as a medical doctor. However, throughout his training, Trager continued to treat people and he was given his own clinic, where he helped those with polio and other neuromuscular problems, with near-miraculous results.

Basically, the therapy of Trager is a form of bodywork that involves gentle stretching, rocking, rolling, bouncing and 'shimmering' (a swift but soft stroking movement over the body). It is extremely soothing for the central nervous system, as the rocking movements take people into a comfort zone, into a very deep state of relaxation. Nothing is forced with Trager, nothing hurts, nothing is remotely uncomfortable or embarrassing. Rather than aiming to go in and fix problems, practitioners try to show the body how it could be more comfortable, more flexible, more easy.

What can trager help?

- It can ease pain and often help to eliminate headaches.
- It promotes greater joint flexibility. The reverberations of the rocking movements echo right through the body and actually massage the internal organs and deep muscles.
- It can help digestion because it tones the abdominal muscles.
- Equally beneficial is Trager's effect on blood circulation, lymphatic drainage and the respiratory system.
- On an emotional level, it battles against stress, eases insomnia and can help you to cope with the strains of modern living.
- Devotees say that Trager gives them a sense of ease and peace, combined with a charge of energy and vitality.

What can I expect from a session?

WHERE WILL I HAVE THE TREATMENT?
You will be lying on a couch.

WILL I BE CLOTHED?
You can wear whatever makes you feel comfortable. Most people eventually end up in underwear, but practitioners will happily work with you fully clothed.

WHAT HAPPENS?
The therapist will first ask a few questions and then ask you to get on the couch. The first movements cradle your head and neck, gently rocking, stretching and flexing. Within minutes, you might find the vertebrae of your neck popping themselves into position quite naturally and painlessly. The session generally floats by like an enchanting dream.

Trager is very different from any other form of bodywork. It does not use the oils or long strokes of conventional massage, nor does it press into the connective tissue as

Rolfing, Hellerwork and Looyenwork do; it does not manipulate the skeletal system as do osteopathy and chiropractic.

WILL IT HURT?
If an area is painful, the last thing a Trager practitioner would do would be to press or prod. Instead, they would back off and try another approach.

WILL ANYTHING STRANGE HAPPEN?
No, you will just experience a delightful feeling of total relaxation.

WILL I BE GIVEN ANYTHING TO TAKE?
No, medication is not part of the treatment.

IS THERE ANY HOMEWORK?
Once you get off the couch, you will be taught a few simple 'exercises', or 'mentastics', as they are known. Not at all arduous nor in any way remotely resembling physical jerks, these exercises are simply little reminders of how to sit, stand and move with ease – ways to continue your Trager session in everyday life. You will be advised to practise these every day for optimum results.

Trager® body awareness

It's nigh-on impossible to duplicate the Trager touch at home. These exercises, however, will help you get a feeling for the Trager philosophy.
• Think about softening, widening, lengthening and expanding. Think about light, lighter and lighter still. Think about a dancing cloud. Now, pause to notice how your body feels as you just think about these things.
• Let one arm drop softly by your side, gently waggle the fingers of your hand and think about feeling the bones. How much does that hand weigh? Now, do the same on the other side. You will probably find that your arms visibly lengthen as you relax.
• Sitting down, imagine that your head is attached to the telling by a large rubber band Feel how that affects your posture – making you straighter, but not bolt upright. Feel your shoulders softly come down, as your head bobs on the rubber band.
• Now imagine that you have a paintbrush fixed to the top of your head and that you are gently painting the ceiling with it. Allow your head to wobble from side to side with slight movements.

17 Energy

Electro-crystal therapy

Electro-crystal therapy doesn't just talk about meridians and chakras; it lets you actually see them. Harry Oldfield, the originator of this remarkable system, is an ex-science teacher who doesn't just tell you about your inner secret-energy self; he lets you see it with your own eyes. Oldfield developed a means of filming the body's subtle energies. While you are scanned with a camera, a multicoloured image of your body appears on a computer screen. On it you can see what mystics have known for years but scientists have refused to admit: energy points (the acupuncture points), energy channels (the meridians), energy centres (the chakras) and the cocooning egg-like field of energy that surrounds us (the aura).

The system is called a poly contrast interface, or PIP, and it is being touted as the X-ray of the future. The camera records very high frequencies of light not normally detected by the human eye. A computer program identifies the waves of light and gives each a different colour reading so that you can literally see the shape of your energy.

Once the problem has been diagnosed, electro-crystal therapy takes over electro magnetic fields are beamed at the patient, using crystals to amplify the energy Oldfield found that, if disease showed up as a disturbance in the body's forcefield, directing a correcting vibratory pattern back into the body would correct the imbalance. However, as he points out, how long the 'cure' lasts depends on the patient.

Oldfield began his healing journey more than 30 years ago with Kirlian photography, when he discovered he could detect illnesses and diseases from the patterns of energy exposed by the photograph. Doctors and scientists were impressed with his findings But when he began to develop more precise diagnostic tools and then to treat – and heal – people, the orthodox community turned away almost en masse. Patients, on the other hand, descended in hordes, their numbers swelling by word-of-mouth Oldfield and his disciples do what very few practitioners of alternative medicine would ever dare do: they talk about remissions and cures for even the most serious and terminal of diseases. To be fair, they don't promise cures and they admit that there are times when people simply don't get well. Even so, they will freely discuss what most people would term miracles.

What can electro-crystal therapy help?

- Practitioners claim it can balance (and hence heal) virtually any disease – some patients have reported nigh-on 'miraculous' recoveries from a wide range of conditions
- People claim to have been cured of eye diseases, degeneration of the optical nerve glaucoma and retinitis pigmentosa.

118

- Some people say mechanical problems with the body have been helped with electro-crystal therapy.
- Children and the elderly seem to respond well.
- Many people use it as a 'last-chance' therapy

What can I expect from a session?

WHERE WILL I HAVE THE TREATMENT?
You will be standing, then sitting, in the practitioner's room.

WILL I BE CLOTHED?
You will be asked to strip to your underwear for the examination. You will be fully clothed for treatment.

WHAT HAPPENS?
The practitioner will move a meter that reads sound waves in the body around you, noting any imbalances. You will then be asked to strip to your underwear while the PIP scanner is pointed at you. You will see yourself on a small computer- screen, your body shape clearly visible, but covered in swirling bands of colour. The practitioner will point out your meridians and chakras, and check your organs and all other parts of your body. A few calculations are then made to work out what frequencies you need for optimum balance. You are next plugged into a small machine while seated in a chair, with a kind of rod pinned under your collarbone and a headband of flexible plastic filled with crystals placed over your head. You sit like this for the whole session.

WILL IT HURT?
Treatment is totally painless – in fact, you don't feel a thing.

WILL ANYTHING STRANGE HAPPEN?
It can be quite strange to see the energy system of your body in such a graphic way. The PIP scanner can pick up imbalances even before they manifest, so you may be given warning of a cold or a sore throat!

WILL I BE GIVEN ANYTHING TO TAKE?
Some practitioners use flower or gem essences in combination with the treatment.

IS THERE ANY HOMEWORK?
Some people buy their own machines for home use, or you may be allowed to borrow one if you need intensive treatment.

Health kinesiology

Health kinesiologists talk to bodies. They bypass the rational mind, preferring to address their questions to the body itself. Give a practitioner of this extraordinary therapy an hour with your body and it will tell him or her exactly what it's allergic to and precisely what is wrong with it, then proceed even to dictate the prescription it requires.

Health kinesiology (HK) was originated by a Canadian scientist, Dr Jimmy Scott. He started out working primarily with allergies. Irritated that most forms of allergy testing were not really accurate, he stumbled upon a system of muscle testing called kinesiology which appeared to be swift, sensitive and reliable. Its principle is that the body, at some deep, unconscious level, knows precisely what it needs. By asking the body directly, the practitioner bypasses the conscious mind, which might think that it knows what is best, but which has really lost touch with the body.

The kinesiologist asks questions by applying light pressure to the patient's outstretched arm while the patient is trying to keep the arm still. If the body answers yes, the arm will resist the pressure and remain strong. If the answer is no, the muscle weakens slightly and the arm will drop. It's rather like dowsing, using the body instead of a pendulum.

Health kinesiology looks at the person as a whole, taking into account their psychological state, their environment, the needs of the physical body and also the interplay between the subtle energy bodies and the chakras (centres of subtle energy in the body). The practitioner will bring the meridian system (lines of subtle energy in the body) into a state of temporary balance before commencing work. Only then, practitioners believe, will muscle testing produce reliable and consistent results. The practitioner then asks the body for permission to continue – to ensure that only appropriate work is done, rather than imposing work on the body. Health kinesiology also uses a variety of highly unusual, and seemingly esoteric, methods for healing the body's imbalances. While the vast majority of scientists and doctors would scoff with cynicism, health kinesiology is not ridiculed in Germany and Switzerland. In these countries, an increasing number of doctors, pharmacists and veterinarians are using this extraordinary therapy as an additional diagnostic tool.

What can health kinesiology help?

- Health kinesiology has helped a seemingly endless array of ailments, including many that have proved immune to other forms of medicine, both orthodox and complementary.
- Practitioners report success with asthma, eczema, migraine, arthritis, acne, menstrual and menopausal problems, irritable bowel syndrome and food allergies.
- As practitioners believe they are working with the body's own healing mechanisms, virtually any complaint is theoretically curable.

What can I expect from a session?

WHERE WILL I HAVE THE TREATMENT?
You will be sitting in the practitioner's therapy room.

WILL I BE CLOTHED?
Yes, you will be fully clothed.

WHAT HAPPENS?
You sit with one arm outstretched while the practitioner talks to your body, asking a long string of questions. They pause almost imperceptibly between each to gauge your arm's response. Once the practitioner has ascertained the problem, as your body perceives it, he or she will ask the body what cures it requires.

Health kinesiology also includes highly unusual techniques for healing, including tapping – touching the body with little tapping movements supposedly clears the body of intolerances and allergies. Sometimes magnets or crystals are placed on the body, homeopathic remedies and essential oils are also held against the body. You might be asked to think of a certain word or phrase while the practitioner holds you.

WILL IT HURT?
No, it's not at all painful.

WILL ANYTHING STRANGE HAPPEN?
Not specifically, but the whole experience feels quite strange.

WILL I BE GIVEN ANYTHING TO TAKE?
Generally, you will just be given the remedy, crystal or oil to hold while the practitioner is working on you, rather than having to take it.

IS THERE ANY HOMEWORK?
Adjustments in lifestyle and diet may be suggested.

Magnetic therapy/alpha pulse therapy

In Japan, magnetic therapy is as mainstream as aspirin. Even the humblest corner store will boast a range of magnetic products – from insoles to car cushions, from back massagers to mattresses. Magnetic therapy may be a multibillion dollar industry, but it's one based on solid scientific research, rather than marketing hype. Clinical trials and studies have shown that using magnetism can have wide-reaching beneficial effects.

The idea that magnets have remarkable properties is nothing new- Cleopatra is said to have worn one on her forehead to keep her beautiful and young. It is only in the past 20 years, however, that the mythology has been proven as medical fact. NASA found that its astronauts were returning to earth feeling sick and debilitated. Intensive research revealed they were suffering withdrawal symptoms from the earth's magnetosphere, which allows the blood to circulate properly and be thoroughly oxygenated. NASA promptly placed static magnets in spacesuits and within the spacecraft, and the problem was overcome. This is known as the Hall Effect – blood flow is stimulated by magnetic pads attracting electrically charged particles (positive and negative ions) in the bloodstream. Even though we generally travel no further than to work and back, many of us suffer a similar problem, albeit on a lesser level. Living in concrete cities, travelling in steel cars, buses, trains and aeroplanes, we are missing out on the health-giving benefits of natural magnetism and so our circulation (and as a consequence, our entire body) Is working under par.

Another type of magnetictherapy is called alpha pulse therapy or pulsed magnetic field (PMF) therapy. This sends very low pulsed fields to the person and has proved extremely effective, particularly for sports injuries and broken bones.

What can magnetic therapy/alpha pulse therapy help?

- Magnets can help boost your general wellbeing, improving sleep and concentration and energy levels, while alleviating stress and tension.
- They are very useful for injuries (aiding recovery of torn muscles, ligaments and tendons, accelerating the healing of bone fractures, and reducing swelling and bruising).
- Alpha pulse therapy, in particular, has had great success with treating osteoporosis.
- They can also ameliorate serious medical conditions (improving mobility in rheumatic and arthritic conditions, easing migraine, correcting hormonal imbalances and treating chronic fatigue).
- Jet lag seems to be diminished and hangovers have been found to disappear after magnetic therapy.
- Some people have discovered that they have mysteriously lost the desire to smoke, while many others have reported that magnetic therapy does wonders for their sex life.
- Alpha pulse therapy seems to be able to treat phobias.

What can I expect from a session?

WHERE WILL I HAVE THE TREATMENT?
You will be lying on a special 'bed' (rather like a sunbed) or, in the case of alpha pulse therapy, on a couch with an arc that transmits the pulsed field over the part requiring treatment.

WILL I BE CLOTHED?
Yes, you will be fully clothed except for shoes and jewellery.

WHAT HAPPENS?
You will be asked if you are pregnant, or have a pacemaker or active cancer (the bed is not suitable for you if any of these apply). You should avoid treatment if you are menstruating or have thrombosis, as it increases blood flow. You then remove shoes and jewellery, and lie down After a few minutes, you may notice some tingling and, after about 15 minutes, the machine tends to become quite warm. Ideally, you would have treatment every day for 10 days. Alpha pulse therapy treatment is similar, but you feel absolutely nothing.

WILL IT HURT?
No, it is totally painless.

WILL ANYTHING STRANGE HAPPEN?
No, although the machine tends to make strange noises and you may notice some tingling. With alpha pulse therapy, you will notice nothing strange.

WILL I BE GIVEN ANYTHING TO TAKE?
No, medication is not part of the treatment.

IS THERE ANY HOMEWORK?
Not specifically, although some people buy equipment (pillows, mattresses, car seats, insoles, bands etc.) for home use.

Polarity therapy

According to polarity therapy, the human body is a living magnet. Just like a magnet, we have electromagnetic currents of energy flowing constantly backwards and forwards within us between positive and negative poles. Polarity therapy teaches that, if we could only regulate an even flow of energy, we would all enjoy rude good health. It's a well-balanced form of natural healthcare, combining nutrition, exercise, bodywork and counselling: a neat synthesis of Eastern and Western therapeutic techniques; a potted, 'best of' complementary therapy.

The founder of polarity therapy was an extraordinary human being called Randolph Stone. Born in 1890, Stone studied a bewildering array of religious philosophies and natural forms of healthcare. He trained as a physician and also learnt osteopathy; chiropractic and naturopathy Sensing that there was still something missing, he then studied Eastern systems of medicine such as ayurveda.

The result of his studies was his conviction that the basis of good health lay purely in energy. Blocked energy was, to his mind, the root cause of all unhappiness and physical illness. It took him 50 years to assemble the comprehensive package that finally became polarity therapy.

Stone taught that energy flows from the centre of any system to its circumference, and then returns by magnetic pull. It will flow from the top downwards, from within the system to without.

A polarity therapist is looking for imbalances in the energy flow which he or she will try to correct using exercise, bodywork, nutrition and counselling.

What can polarity therapy help?

- Polarity therapy usually manages to improve most conditions.
- It has consistently good results with migraine, digestive problems and allergies.
- Myalgic encephalomyelitis (ME) and other debilitating illnesses respond well, as do all stress-related illnesses,
- Back pain and sciatica generally improve or are cured with polarity therapy.
- It's excellent if you feel you need to get back in touch with your body and need an overall grounding in healthy living.

What can I expect from a session?

WHERE WILL I HAVE THE TREATMENT?
You will be in the therapist's room: lying on a couch for bodywork; sitting in chairs for nutritional guidance and counselling; on the floor for polarity yoga.

WHAT HAPPENS?
You will be asked to monitor your diet for 5 days before your first session, simply writing down everything you eat and drink. You will then spend some time in the first session talking about your life, health and any problems. You will then be asked to sit on a chair or lie on a couch. The touch is firm and focused, pressing deeply into points of tension and manipulating stiff joints. You may also find yourself being rocked or shaken to stimulate energy flow.

Afterwards, you will be given dietary guidelines, often cleansing diets or juice fasts. Time is set aside just to talk – emotional wellbeing is seen as essential.

Finally, you will be taught some polarity yoga exercises – simple poses which are held either statically or while gently rocking.

WILL I BE CLOTHED?
Yes, unless you have a structural problem that is clearer with you undressed.

WILL IT HURT?
Some points can feel quite tender, but generally it doesn't hurt and is very relaxing.

WILL I BE GIVEN ANYTHING TO TAKE?
Medication is not a part of the treatment, but you will probably be given dietary guidelines.

IS THERE ANY HOMEWORK?
Yes, lots. Expect to be asked to shift your eating habits and also to practice polarity yoga. You may be advised to go on a juice fast or cleansing diet.

Do-it-yourself polarity therapy

THE PURIFYING DIET
This diet is said to help constipation, high blood pressure, arthritis and rheumatism, congestion and general toxicity. Try it for a weekend to begin with. While on this regime, cut out all dairy produce, tea and coffee, alcohol, carbohydrates and starchy foods. Water can be drunk freely. If you have any health concerns, check with your doctor before carrying out this diet.

First thing – two or more cups of hot herbal tea made from equal amounts of liquorice root, anise or fennel, peppermint and fenugreek. Add fresh ginger, lemon juice and honey to taste.

Breakfast – liver-flush juice: 3-4 tablespoons of pure cold-pressed olive or almond oil with twice the amount of fresh lemon juice. Add 3-6 cloves crushed garlic, plus fresh ginger to taste.

Mid-morning (two hours after breakfast) – 225 ml/8 fl oz of fresh vegetable juice, made from cabbage, lettuce, carrot and beetroot. Add radish or onion if you like and ginger, lemon, honey and garlic to taste.

Lunch (noon) – raw salad of fresh radish, lettuce, cabbage, grated carrot, onion, cucumber, tomato and sprouts You may use a little dressing of almond, olive or sesame oil with lemon, garlic, onion and ginger. Fresh fruit for dessert. Mid-afternoon – as for midmorning. Evening meal (around 6 pm) – fruit: choose from apples, pears, grapes, pomegranate and papaya Herbal tea. If you are very hungry, you may repeat the lunchtime salad.

JUICING FOR HEALTH
Polarity therapy strongly advocates the use of fresh, organic fruit and vegetable juices to help the healing process. Try out the combinations given below (equal quantities of each ingredient, taken freely) for the following common conditions:

Anxiety and nervous tension – lemon and lime

Arthritis – carrot, celery and cabbage

Asthma and catarrh – carrot and radish

Low blood pressure – carrot, beetroot and dandelion

Blocked sinuses – horseradish and lemon (use 100 g/4 oz horseradish and 50 ml/2 fl oz lemon juice, combined with a teaspoon of garlic juice and a tablespoon of honey – take a teaspoon four times daily)

Constipation – cabbage, spinach, celery and lemon

Insomnia – celery

Skin conditions – carrot, beetroot and celery

Sore throats and colds – lemon, lime and pineapple

Radionics

Radionics has been dubbed the medicine of the future and, at first glance, it seems like nothing more than science fiction. Say you need to consult your doctor, but you are in Australia on business while your doctor is in the UK. You simply ring him, explain your symptoms, put down the telephone and wait. Back in the UK, your doctor takes out your file and scans a sample of hair you provided several years ago. Popping it in a machine, he directs a light beam through a series of cards for a few minutes. End of treatment. Some 17,000 km (10,000 miles) away, you start to feel better. Wishful thinking? Apparently not.

Radionic systems of healing have been in use since the early part of the twentieth century. Practitioners worked with a pendulum to find their diagnosis and remedy, by means of a process of dowsing. In addition, they employed curious 'black boxes' which measured what they then believed were simply electromagnetic forces. Until recently, however, they were generally dismissed as quacks, with diagnosis and cures summoned seemingly by the practitioner's supposed psychic powers influencing the pendulum.

Radionics, however, has lately taken on a fresh lease of life, having been given credibility with new advances in physics. Quantum physicists perceive nothing odd or alien about a system of medicine that takes no notice of time or place; that ignores physical examination and doesn't need to treat you with pills or potions.

Illness, according to the radionic consultant, occurs when there is a disturbance to our energetic frequency. It's rather as though we were radio stations – the signal sometimes gets a little confused and you need to twiddle the radio dial a bit.

What can radionics help?

- Satisfied customers claim they have been cured of a wide variety of ailments, including asthma, eczema, irritable bowel syndrome and chronic fatigue, to name but a few.
- Some doctors, dentists and specialists refer cases that orthodox techniques can't help.

What can I expect from a session?

WHERE WILL I HAVE THE SESSION?
Initial sessions are usually held at the therapist's consulting room. You will be seated in a chair.

WILL I BE CLOTHED
Yes, you will be fully clothed.

WHAT HAPPENS?
A radionics case history will include not only questions about past illnesses and operations, but also about your hobbies and pastimes, and even your temperament. You will be asked for a small piece of hair, which acts as a 'witness', a way of tuning in to your vibration. Your hair will remain in energetic equilibrium with its source and its energetic characteristics will vary from moment to moment according to your own energetic patterns. If you can accept this (and it does take a radical shift in thinking), it becomes logical (if not perhaps understandable) that correcting imbalances of energy within the hair witness will set up a ripple effect and bring the rest of the patient back into balance.

Radionics practitioners don't rely solely on such subtle means of energetic healing. Sometimes they send people back to their doctors with an accurate diagnosis, or they refer to dentistry, as radionics theory recognizes is a firm link between general health and the teeth. There may be dietary solutions or the person may be referred to an osteopath because of a mechanical problem.

WILL IT HURT?
No, not at all.

WILL ANYTHING STRANGE HAPPEN?
Frankly, the whole radionics experience is strange!

WILL I BE GIVEN ANYTHING TO TAKE?
You may be referred to a homeopath or given flower remedies.

IS THERE ANY HOMEWORK?
You may need to have further consultations with other specialists, once a firm diagnosis has been obtained.

Index

Acknowledgements

I certainly could not have written this book single-handedly – so I would like to give heartfelt thanks to the many experts who have given so generously their time and knowledge to me. They include: Angela Hope-Murray, Judith Morrison, Doja Purkitt, Dr Rajendra Sharma, Andrew Johnson, Ruth Delman and Kenneth Gibbons, Dr Tamara Voronina, Roger Newman Turner, Dr Andrew Lockie, Roger Savage, Penelope Ritchie, Keith and Chrissie Mason, Kate Roddick, Rosalie Samet, Dr Natsagdorj, Karin Weisensel, Dr Mohammad Salim Khan, Linda Lazarides, Patrick Holford, Dr Marilyn Glenville, Fiona Arrigo, Nicola Griffin, Andrew Chevalier, Christine Steward, Godfrey Devereux, Sebastian Pole, Charlotte Katz, Sue Weston, Malcolm Kirsch, Joel Carbonnel, Kate Kelly, Gail Barlow, Barbara McCrea, Julie Crocker, Jane Thurnell-Read, Geraint and Sylvia Jones-David, Wilma Tait, Tom Williams, Sarah Shurety, Liz Williams, Simon Brown, William Spear, Karen Kingston, Denise Linn, Gina Lazenby, Kajal Sheth, Lynne Crawford, Rob Russell, Kati Cottrell-Blanc, Jane Mayers, Richard Lanham, Ron Wilgosh, Dave Hawkes, Jo Hogg, Kieran Foley, Jennie Crewdson, Terry Peterson, Allan Rudolf, Carol Logan, Tony Bailey, Angela Renton, Gillie Gilbert, Sarah Dening, Patricia Martello, Gabrielle Roth, Caroline Born, Shan, Leo Rutherford, Kenneth Meadows, Howard Charing, William Bloom, Will Parfitt, Vera Diamond, Maria Mercati, Julian Baker, Monica Anthony, Phil Parker, Jon Mason, Jeff Leonard, Peter Bartlett, Corina Petter, Sue Ricks, Pat Morrell, Rosalyn Journeaux, Elaine Arthey, Pim de Gryff, Sara Hooley, Eileen Fairbane, Dee Jones, Jessica Loeb, Emma Field, Narendra Mehta, Jill Dunley, Agni Eckroyd, Harry Oldfield, Rosamund Webster, Margaret-Anne Pauffley and Paul Dennis, Natalie Handley, Chris James, Susan Lever, Angelika Hochadel, Gaston Saint-Pierre.

Lots of love to the original Williams family who started me off on this curious path and to the many friends and fellow seekers who have guided me along the way.

A large debt of gratitude to Bonnie Estridge who introduced me to Carlton Books and to everyone there.

A big hug as always to über-agent Judy Chilcote.